A CHILD WILL LEAD
KIDS OF ALL AGES™

BY
MAX STURMAN

Author of

Never Get a Cold
No Sugar No Flour Will Give ME the Power
Do It Naturally

This is a nonprofit venture.
That's it! Pure and simple.
There is no solicitation of any kind,
and you may reproduce anything in this book.

Give this book to someone who will benefit
from this information. Pass it along!

HEALTH IS THE ONLY TRUE WEALTH.

Published by
Do it Naturally Foundation
msturman@san.rr.com
5236 Cole St
San Diego, CA 92117

© 2009, Max Sturman
ISBN: 0-9770674-6-6

Printed in the United States of America
10 9 8 7 6 5 4 3 2 1

Disclaimer: This book is for information and educational purposes only. The author and publisher recommend you consult your health care advisor before starting any diet or making a lifestyle change.

Table of Contents

7   Acknowledgments

9   This Book is to be Read by Kids of All Ages

12 Complications of Childhood Obesity

13 Mexico is second-fattest nation AFTER U.S.(News article)

17 Obesity / BMI chart

18 Alzheimer's Disease and the Latino Community

21 Arthritis

22 Diabetes Treatments Under Fire

24 Japan measuring waistlines to rein in growth in obesity

26 Your car gets better care than your body

28 Owner's Manual

29 Success will come

30 Choosing to make America healthier

33 The Immune System

35 Fast facts

36 Portion, serving sizes are different

37 Meal Portions Today Compared to 20 years ago

38 Nutrition Fact Labels

40 What Are You Drinking?

41 Diet Drinks—Aspartame

43 Energy Drinks

45 Healthy Drinks?

47 Steering teens away from drugs, alcohol (news article)

49 Binge Drinking proves deadly for more college-age victims

51 Food Additives

Table of Contents

52   Supplement called "fountain of youth"

54   Analysts see business of candy as recession-proof

57   Wheaty Indiscretions

63   No-Nos! and Okay Foods

64   Bad Food Choices/ Good Food Choices

65   General Eating Guidelines

66   What is Fiber?

68   Companies Sued for Carcinogens in Food

69   For the Children

70   Center for Science in the Public Interest

73   Exercise Before and After

74   One exercise fits all? "Not by any stretch"

77   Why Did Tim Die?

78   Evolution

79   144 Reasons Why Sugar Is Ruining Your Health

85   The Eight Essential Biological Sugars

86   The Top 20 Worst Restaurant Foods in America

88   Nature's Design

89   Take these steps to cut diabetes risk

91   Watermelon

93   Secret's in the Sauce

94   Could *hot cocoa* be the next "wonder drug" for high blood pressure?

95   Cholesterol drugs advised for kids with risk factors

97   Conclusions for a Healthy Life

98   What is happiness?

99   About the author

Acknowledgments

As with any major project, its completion is contingent upon the giving nature of many people — made even more poignant with a non-profit venture, such as this book. There are many who have contributed to *You Are What You Eat, Dude!* Some in more pronounced ways than others, but certainly no less important.

Although I have tried to include the names here, of those whose dedication and assistance in the writing of this book is truly appreciated, there is always someone whose name misses the credits — you know, like forgetting your spouse's contribution when accepting an Oscar. So if you are one who made a contribution to *You Are What You Eat, Dude!* and your name does not appear in these credits, please accept my apology and feel free to contact me. I'll make sure you're added for the next printing!

To these fine people, I offer my heartfelt thanks: Carlos and Julie and her staff at Paradise Printing (San Diego); my editors on this project Ariana Zahedi; LinDee Rochelle ; Nancy Appleton; Andrea Glass; Dr. Dennis Goodman MD; Jan Harris; Trish Hinkley; Sharon Thomerson (Librarian); DDK, Fazi Salooti, Sylvia Auerbach, Jacobs Family Service; and all of the reporters and publications who wrote and published the various articles included in this book, or from which I excerpted information.

James Hervey Johnson Charitable Educational Trust

THIS BOOK IS TO BE READ BY KIDS OF ALL AGES

There must be something wrong with our society when there are conditions in this world that cause the epidemic diseases prevalent today. But it wasn't like this in primitive times, when the lifestyle was far different, with an entirely different diet and activity needs.

Even in this day and age, there are countries where the "SAD" (Standard American Diet) has not invaded their way of eating. People have lived without any of the degenerative diseases and in vital health, even into their hundreds.

Apparently, we need a change in our educational system to teach the children, parents, teachers, dieticians and, oh yes, the educators. They need vital information on how to take proper care of our bodies and to eliminate once and for all those harmful foods and the lifestyle that have caused all this damage.

> ### *This book, then, is an attempt to reverse the trend we're in.*

A good way to start is to teach our children the mantra ...

NO SUGAR NO FLOUR WILL GIVE **ME** THE POWER

This chant is an easy one to remember for even the smallest child … and when told to the parents … will send a message and plea to provide healthy food for the child, *and* for the parents!

"Mommy, I'm tired of getting colds, and earaches, and having a sick tummy, especially when I can't go out and play with my friends, and have to stay in bed all day. When I don't go to school, I miss a lot. Also, I don't like having to make up the school work I miss. Also, I don't like taking that awful tasting stuff that the doctor says will make me better — but it takes such a long time! Mommy, why do people have to get sick? I want to be all better again and feel good!"

People didn't always get sick. Primitive man was a hunter and gatherer. The lifestyle at the time required much effort and energy to live, and to sustain life. The food supply was what was grown in the earth and the meat from the animals in the wild. Nature provided abundantly all that was needed to survive. The people were strong and healthy, and even though they had a hard life, they didn't have the diseases we have in our modern society.

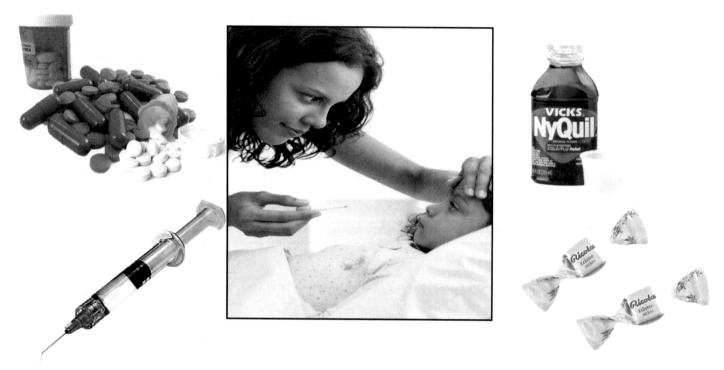

Children don't want to be sick. They want to be healthy. Understanding the direct effect food has on your body and therefore making informed choices of what you put into it, is the secret to being healthy. In this day of an overabundance of food choices, it is imperative that we understand the nutrition fact labels, lists of ingredients, and serving sizes, as well as percentage daily values required. Because these labels are listed in grams, one needs to know the conversion to the American measuring system (tbs., tsp., etc.).

Processed sugar is an addictive, harmful ingredient in many of our foods, even foods that we would never suspect. Sugar is listed under several names; one must be alert to this. We are told that artificial sweeteners are "safe" because they have been tested and approved by the FDA (Food & Drug Administration); but there is still much controversy as to their safety. Artificial sweeteners have been linked with neurological diseases, such as Alzheimer's.

Let's take a look at a soda, something lots of people drink every day. Each soda has 40 grams of sugar; this equals 10 teaspoons of sugar, and that's a lot! Beverage companies have been alerted to this and have begun to reduce the amount of sugar. But we must be careful to read the nutrition facts and ingredient labels to get a true understanding of what the product contains. Does this change make the soda a healthful, nutritious drink?

Water is your best choice for a healthful, nutritious drink! Freshly-squeezed fruit and vegetable juices are also healthy. Too much juice would not be good for some people who have certain conditions, such as diabetes, Candida, etc. You are better off with freshly-squeezed juices rather than processed juices, which contain preservatives. Again, water is your best choice. Tap water has been tested and processed for safety, and is considered safe.

The United States and Mexico are the fattest nations in the world. In Mexico where hunger once prevailed, diabetes is now the leading cause of death. According to the latest national surveys, more than 71% of Mexican women, 66% of Mexican men, and a quarter of Mexican children ages 5 to 11, are overweight. This is found to be directly attributed to the rising popularity of soft drinks and fast foods restaurants. Foods that were once unavailable, both healthy and unhealthy, can now be purchased at modern supermarkets.

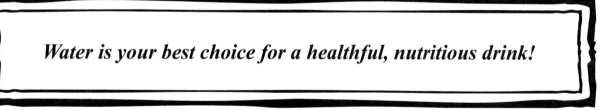

Water is your best choice for a healthful, nutritious drink!

In some parts of Mexico it is easier to get a soda, than a clean glass of water. In the past 14 years, the consumption of soft drinks has increased 60%! Legislators have considered putting warning labels on junk food but have met great resistance from powerful industry groups. Leaders hope that the growing concern over diabetes will lead to greater public acceptance of the association of sugar with diabetes. More than 70,000 Mexicans now die each year from diabetes-related conditions, and it is now the leading cause of death in that country.

Mexico is just an example of what can happen to the population of a country when junk becomes part of the national diet. But it's not alone — the U.S. has the most obese population; Mexico is in second place. Obesity is a worldwide problem.

Complications of Childhood Obesity

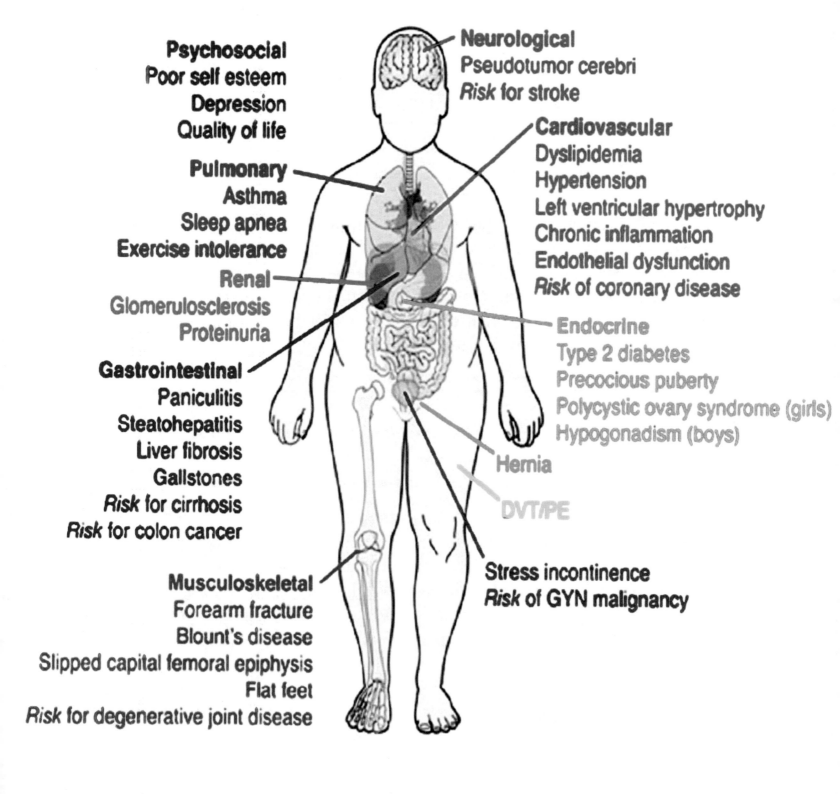

Mexico is second-fattest nation AFTER U.S.

"Where hunger once prevailed, diabetes is leading cause of death"

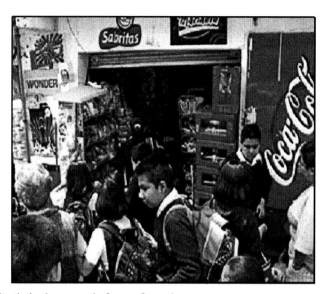

By Franco Ordonez
ICT News Service/*San Diego Union-Tribune*
March 24, 2008

MEXICO CITY — Fueled by the rising popularity of soft drinks and fast food restaurants, Mexico has become the second-fattest nation in the world. Mexican health officials say it could surpass the United States as the most obese country within 10 years if trends continue.

More than 71 percent of Mexican women and 66 percent of Mexican men are overweight, according to the latest national surveys.

With diabetes now Mexico's leading cause of death, activists and leaders hope to renew efforts to crack down on fatty-food consumption and encourage citizens to exercise more. But it will be a tough battle, as industry groups are expected to put up a fight. No one knows better the country's affection for fattening foods than Lidia Garcia Garduno, who's run a fruit stand in central Mexico City for the past 10 years.

People don't eat right anymore," said Garcia Garduno, mixing a drink of strawberries and pineapple. "Instead of coming here and purchasing a fruit drink, they prefer to walk across the street and buy fried pork chips. That's why so many Mexicans are obese."

In 1989, fewer than 10 percent of Mexican adults were overweight. No one in the country even talked about obesity back then, said Barry Popkin, a University of North Carolina-Chapel Hill professor who studies global weight gain. Experts were too concerned with poverty and hunger.

"It certainly snuck up on them," said Popkin, who's working with the Mexican health ministry to develop strategies to address obesity throughout the country. "Mexico has probably had the most rapid increase of obesity in the last 15 years."

Mexican Health Secretary Jose Cordova, who launched a new health campaign Feb. 25, agrees: "We have to put the brakes on this obesity problem."

Some Mexicans say there's less space on an already crowded Mexico City subway because riders are getting larger. At a flea market in the south of the city, vendors hawk clothes brought from the United States made for overweight individuals.

Francisco Princegali knew he was eating too much junk food when he bent down last week and heard a tear. "I ripped my pants because of the fat," said Princegali, who's 20, crumbling up a wrapper of sweetened bread he'd purchased from a vendor. "I think I'm addicted to junk food." Princegali, sucking in his stomach, said many of his pants were too tight these days. Some people are addicted to alcohol and smoking, he said: "My problem is I love fried chicken — Kentucky Fried Chicken."

As in the United States, Mexicans are living more sedentary lives. Studies show that they're eating more fat and processed foods and fewer whole grains and vegetables. Foods — healthy and unhealthy — that once were unavailable now can be purchased at modern supermarkets. In some areas of the country, it's easier to get a soft drink than a clean glass of water. The vast majority of Mexico City's public schools, and many private schools, lack drinkable water, Popkin said.

The national study also found that a quarter of Mexican children ages 5 to 11 are too heavy, a 40 percent increase since 2000.

According to the government's National Institute of Public Health, the consumption of soft drinks increased 60 percent in Mexico over the past 14 years.

st week, children lined up to purchase soft drinks and potato chips outside their school in the
nter of Mexico City.

rginia Soriano, 35, said it was difficult teaching her children good eating habits when they were
oded with advertising for fatty foods. Naomi, her daughter, said her favorite things to eat are
cDonald's Chicken McNuggets and Coca-Cola. The 6 year old sometimes pushes away her
nner plate if it has too many vegetables, Soriano said.

he'll say, 'This has no taste,'" Soriano said. "She wants McDonald's or Kentucky Fried
icken."

gislators have considered putting warning labels on junk food and taxing whole milk to
courage consumption of skim milk. Past efforts have foundered, however, and some lawmakers
ve reported difficulty fighting powerful industry groups. In 2006, legislators voted down a
oposed tax on soft drinks, arguing that it discriminated against the poor. Leaders hope that the
owing concern over diabetes will lead to greater public acceptance of such efforts.

psiCo joined the education ministry last year in launching a new health program, "Living
althily," that encourages more daily exercise and better eating habits. But consumer group El
der del Consumidor, "Power of the Consumer," has accused the company of surreptitiously
arketing its products to children.

onica Bauer, a spokeswoman for PepsiCo International, said that the program, which includes a
deo game that teaches healthy eating habits, didn't include any advertising.

Ve understand there is an obesity problem," she said. "We're trying to be part of the solution."

The health consequences of obesity include increased rates of diabetes, high blood pressure and heart disease. The Mexican Diabetes Federation estimates that 6.5 million to 10 million Mexicans have diabetes.

More than 70,000 Mexicans die each year from diabetes-related conditions, Cordova said. He said that the diabetes burden was draining Mexico's already strained health services and that if trends continued, the country's health care system would be bankrupt within a decade.

"If we don't stop this, we're going to run out of money to treat the sick," Cordova said.

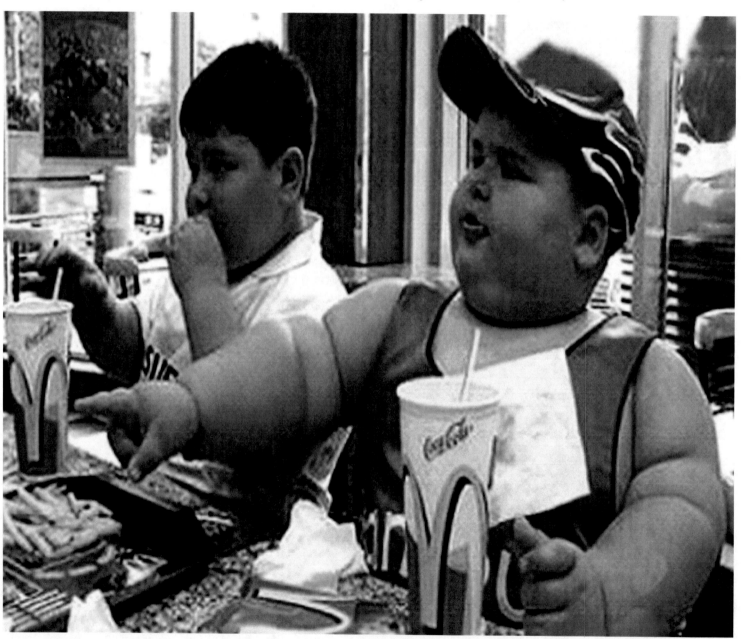

OBESITY:
The percentage of the population older than 15 with a body-mass index greater than 30.

Female

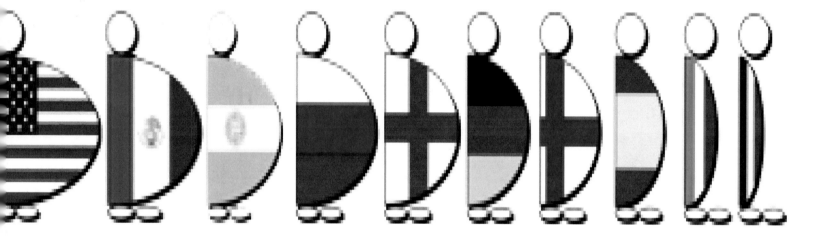

Male

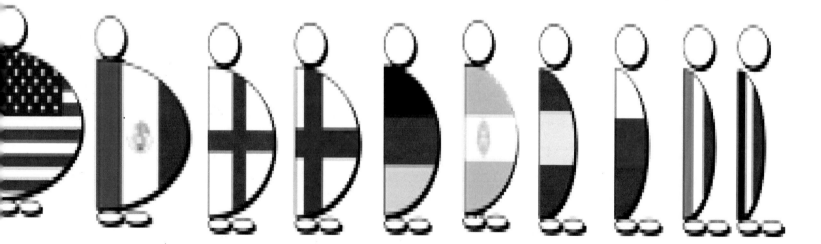

...here are many variables, but the average, healthy 15-year-old-boy for instance, should have a BMI (Body Mass Index) of approximately 23-25.

...epartment of Health & Human Services, www.cdc.gov.)

"Alzheimer's Disease and the Latino Community"

By Ed Martinez
San Diego Union-Tribune
May 2, 2008

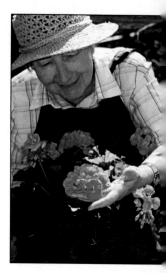

The Salk Institute and the University of California San Diego recently published a study that found some of the factors that cause diabetes might also trigger Alzheimer's. This only dramatizes the "Alzheimer's tsunami" faced by the Latino community.

Recent data from the Centers for Disease Control and Prevention show that this group develops diabetes at twice the rate of the general population. The similarities between a tsunami and Alzheimer's are noteworthy: both often evolve undetected and strike their victims without warning; both result in great loss of human life and cause extreme distress for loved ones and families; and both require a high state of community awareness and preparedness to minimize future losses.

Latinos are now the fastest-growing population in the United States and are generally considered to be at higher risk for developing Alzheimer's disease due to three factors: (1) an increasing life expectancy with an average age of 87 by 2050; (2) higher rates of cardiovascular risk factors such as diabetes and high blood pressure; and (3) lower utilization of available health services.

According to the National Institute on Aging, Alzheimer's disease and related dementias among Latinos are projected to increase more than 600 percent in the United States during the first half of the 21st century. This increase, a looming tsunami, means that 1.3 million Latinos will have Alzheimer's by 2050, compared with fewer than 200,000 currently living with the disease.

Based on these alarming estimates from public health demographers, community health advocates fear that unprepared and unsuspecting Latino communities are currently vulnerable to an epidemic of Alzheimer's disease that could strike with the power of a destructive tsunami.

It is a daunting challenge to prepare the Latino community for a thunderous wave of this proportion — particularly since local safety net providers already work so hard to provide health care services to thousands of elderly, at-risk Latinos, many of whom already have symptoms of Alzheimer's disease and other related dementia.

Based on the following challenges facing our Latino community, we strongly believe that the tsunami-like characteristics of this disease will gradually engulf the community's capacity to maintain the health and well-being of its elderly residents:

In 2000, about 1,900 elderly Latinos with Alzheimer's lived in San Diego. The Alzheimer's Association San Diego/Imperial Chapter recently reported that in the South Bay there are currently 9,012 elderly Latinos at risk for Alzheimer's disease, and by 2050 the prevalence of Alzheimer's among Latinos in San Diego County is estimated to increase to 23,300 — an alarming increase of 1,233 percent.

Elderly Latinos report lower utilization of medical services due to language/communication problems and cultural misunderstandings. These access barriers often lead to higher levels of physical impairment due to delays in early diagnosis and treatment. Without adequate (new) resources to expand the availability of culturally competent health and social support services, elderly Latinos at-risk for Alzheimer's disease will continue to underutilize institutional-based programs offering diagnostic and treatment services.

The situation clearly is urgent. Yet, despite the ominous swell of the Alzheimer's tsunami charging toward the Latino community, governmental and nongovernmental entities have allocated only limited resources for community-based preventive, diagnostic and treatment services.

However, in 2004, the Alzheimer's Association received a three-year grant from The California Endowment to establish a pilot dementia care network targeting the South Bay's Latino community. San Ysidro Health Center and Casa Familiar collaborated with the Alzheimer's Association in implementing community-based dementia care services, including community outreach and health education, family counseling, recreational activities and health care referrals for
diagnosis and medical treatment.

In addition, in early 2006, Supervisor Greg Cox's Office funded a one-year community outreach program sponsored by the Alzheimer's Association. This initiative focused on the South Bay community and was designed to raise the Latino community's awareness of Alzheimer's and related dementias.

Although these two funding programs were of limited scope, they proved to be very successful in demonstrating the effectiveness of public-private partnerships in developing and implementing community-based Alzheimer's services. Given the urgency of maintaining essential risk-reduction, early diagnosis and primary care services for at-risk elderly Latinos, we have agreed to continue funding the dementia care network on a limited basis until additional funding is secured.

The Latino community also supports the Alzheimer's Association effort to increase federal funding for Alzheimer's research at $1 billion per year. This level of funding would help support the association's research program and expand its efforts to better understand long-standing access barriers in the Latino community that delay early diagnosis and treatment.

Clearly, we can only prepare for this Alzheimer's tsunami that is bearing down on the Latino community through collaboration, networking and leveraging of scarce resources.

* * * * * * * * * * * * * * * * * * *

Martinez, a physician, is chief executive officer of the San Ysidro Health Center.

Arthritis

There are many forms of arthritis. Some experience pain in joints, stiffness, inflammation, swelling, fatigue and chronic pain. Depression caused by inability to be normally active, is always evident.

The Arthritis Foundation offers a variety of fitness classes featuring various exercises that are specifically programmed for arthritic patients. Daily exercise is recommended. The importance of doing these exercises is a *must* to help in recovery, but it doesn't have to be hard.

Arthritis is a diet-related disease, and the first thing one must do, is stop doing what caused it in the first place!

To improve your arthritis: Make a complete change to the appropriate diet, avoiding harmful chemical additives, together with a daily exercise program.

You can look forward to a complete recovery, if you have not waited too long. In advanced cases supervised fasting has produced remarkable, positive results.

THIS WAS A OLDER PERSON'S DISEASE, BUT NOW YOUNGER PEOPLE ARE GETTING IT!

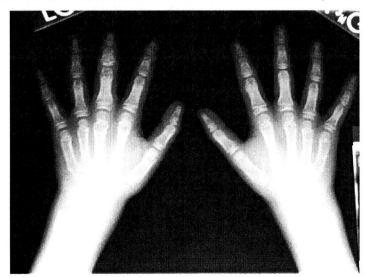

Arthritis is a diet-related disease, and the first thing one must do, is stop doing what caused it in the first place!

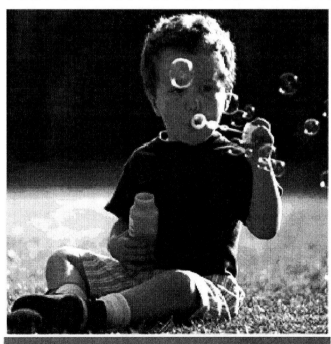

The systemic type of juvenile arthritis usually starts in children under 5.

Diabetes Treatments Under Fire

To show that we must examine every side to an issue or story, below is an article that discusses two decidedly different studies conducted on the affects of obesity on diabetes sufferers, producing opposite results!

Add to this, the devastating truth that more children are overweight and diagnosed with diabetes than ever before. As with many diseases, we know a lot about how and why diabetes occurs, but there is new evidence that a diabetes link to heart disease may change some current treatment practices.

"The diabetes and obesity epidemics"

By Steven V. Edelman
(UCSD professor of medicine and founder, Taking Control of Your Diabetes)
San Diego Union-Tribune **(condensed)**
June 12, 2008

Diabetes affects tens of millions of people in the United States and costs about $174 billion each year in medical expenditures — more than any other health condition. Even worse, diabetes is the sixth leading cause of death in the United States. There is no way to measure the enormous amount of suffering that goes along with this condition.

… After exploring the benefits of aggressively lowering blood glucose in patients with type 2 diabetes and heart disease, the studies came to very similar conclusions but with different effects. While both demonstrated that aggressive glucose control did not have any benefit on reducing heart disease, the National Institutes of Health's study found that **some people with diabetes who dramatically lowered their blood glucose levels actually had more fatal heart attacks than those who didn't.**

… On the other hand, the second study, conducted by the George Institute for International Health in Australia, found no evidence of an increased risk of death among type 2 diabetes patients receiving intensive treatment to lower their blood glucose levels. In fact, these patients were actually found to have a 20 percent reduced risk for kidney disease as a result of the treatment.

.. Though differing opinions abound, one thing is clear: the diabetes treatment paradigm is poised for much needed change.

Managing blood sugar levels alone to treat diabetes is no longer good enough. ... we need to individualize treatment and address the underlying cause of type 2 diabetes and its associated conditions in order to improve patient health.

.. We know that excess weight exacerbates health problems like high blood pressure and abnormal cholesterol levels in diabetes patients, often leading to heart disease and kidney failure, among other problems.

.. managing weight is critical for people who have diabetes or are at risk for developing diabetes. Despite the mounting evidence supporting the synergistic benefits of lowering blood glucose levels and weight in patients with type 2 diabetes, **weight management is not routinely addressed as part of the treatment paradigm.** In fact, many of the diabetes medications most often prescribed by doctors actually cause patients to gain weight. Focusing on both glucose control and obesity when treating type 2 diabetes is of vital importance.

Patients need to understand their own roles in lowering both weight and blood glucose. ... At a minimum, patients should be referred to dietitians, exercise specialists or certified diabetes educators.

Once patients and health care professionals begin working together to manage all aspects of diabetes, we'll see more patients achieving a much better standard of care. This means many San Diegans and other Americans with diabetes can live healthier, happier and more productive lives.

* * * * * * * * * * * * * * * * * * * *

"Japan measuring waistlines to rein in growth in obesity"

By Norimitsu Onishi
New York Times News Service/*San Diego Union-Tribune*
June 13, 2008

Amagasaki, Japan – Japan, a country not known for its overweight people, has undertaken one of the most ambitious campaigns ever by a nation to slim down its citizenry.
Summoned by the city of Amagasaki one recent morning, flower shop owner Minoru Nogiri, 45 found himself lining up to have his waistline measured. With no visible paunch, he seemed to run little risk of being classified as overweight, or *metabo,* the preferred word in Japan these days.

But because the new state-prescribed limit for male waistlines was 33.5 inches, he had anxiously measured himself at home a couple of days earlier. "I'm on the border," he said.
Under a national law that came into effect two months ago, companies and local governments must measure the waistlines of Japanese people between the ages of 40 and 74 as part of their annual checkups. That represents more than 56 million waistlines, or about 44 percent of the population.

Those exceeding government limits – 33.5 inches for men and 35.4 inches for women, the thresholds established in 2005 for Japan by the International Diabetes Federation as an easy guideline for identifying health risks – and suffering from a weight-related ailment will be given dieting guidance if after three months they do not lose weight. If necessary, those people will be steered toward further re-education after six more months.

To reach its goals of shrinking the overweight population by 10 percent over the next four years and 25 percent over the next seven years, the government will impose financial penalties on companies and local governments that fail to meet specific targets.

The country's Ministry of Health argues that the campaign will keep the spread of strokes and diseases such as diabetes in check.

The ministry also says that curbing widening waistlines will rein in a rapidly aging society's ballooning health care costs, one of the most serious and politically delicate problems facing Japan today.

Most Japanese are covered under public health care or through their work. Anger over a plan that would make those 75 and older pay more for health care recently brought a parliamentary censure motion against Prime Minister Yasuo Fukuda, the first against a prime minister in the country's postwar history.

But critics say that the government guidelines – especially the one about male waistlines – are too strict and that more than half of all men will be considered overweight. The effect, they say, will be to encourage overmedication and ultimately raise health care costs.

Yoichi Ogushi, a professor at Tokai University's School of Medicine near Tokyo, said that there was "no need at all" for the Japanese to lose weight.

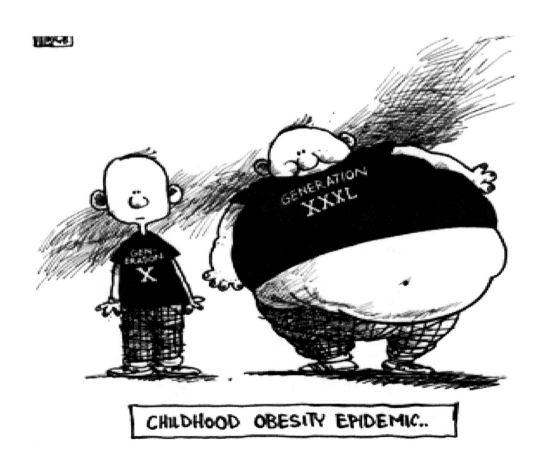

CHILDHOOD OBESITY EPIDEMIC..

Our family just bought a new car, and what a beauty it is. You just know
we are going to baby it and take good care and maintain it,
because it has to last us a long time.

Your car gets better care than your body

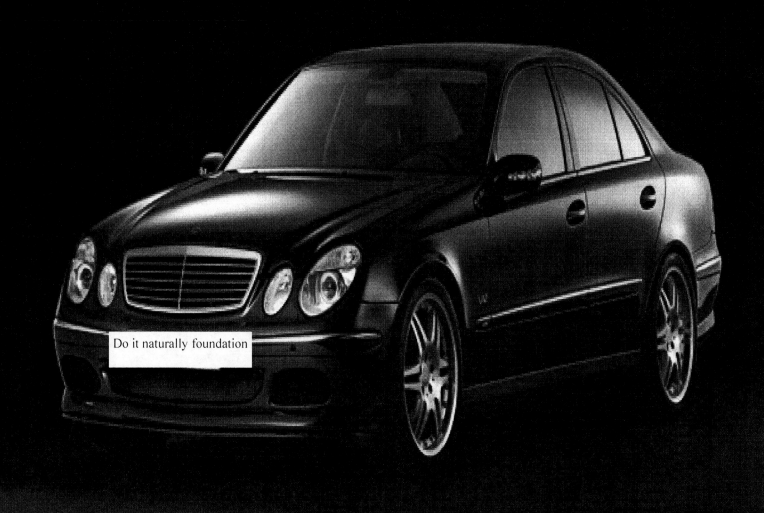

Do it naturally foundation

The car comes with an owner's manual and we have read it thoroughly and intend to do all the necessary oil changes at 3,000 miles, check all fluids and make sure it is reliable and in tip top shape. We will use the appropriate gas, oils and water as needed. In other words we will take meticulous care of the car.

Now, why don't we take care of our bodies just as seriously? We wouldn't *think* of putting garbage in our precious car, so why do we put it in our bodies?

It just doesn't make much sense that we take better care of our cars than we do our bodies. We keep putting in all kinds of harmful foods that make us sick, when we need the right foods that make us well; when we need the right food for proper nutrition to give us optimum performance.

We are bombarded with advertisements through television, radio, magazines and newspapers. They mercilessly give us the message that induce us to buy their products. Unfortunately the junk food in our society is addictive, and it is very difficult to break the habit. Many who try, have withdrawal symptoms and fail.

Change your eating habits and you change your life.

> *It just doesn't make much sense that we take better care of our cars than we do our bodies.*

Owner's Manual

To get maximum performance it is recommended you do not use other than suggested fuel. Any deviation will void this warranty and result in serious damage and eventual breakdown.

Fuel: all fresh fruits and vegetables, nuts, whole grains.

DO NOT OVERFILL
Meats, fats, dairy, eggs, fish … as needed.

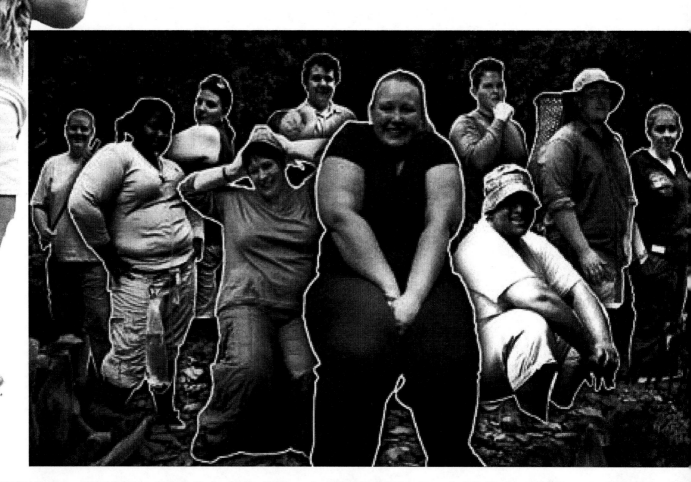

EXTENDED WARRANTY AVAILABLE

Success Will Come!

Success will come:
When those who have the discipline and information to lick
the obesity obstacle return to good health.

Success will come:
With education regarding our national needs.

Success will come:
When we pass legislation that will clarify nutritional fact labels
and lists of ingredients.

Success will come:
When these items will be in language we can understand.

Success will come:
When the marketplace will have only healthy foods.

Success will come:
When harmful foods are exposed for what they are.

Success will come:
When exercise will be a prime priority and
TV, VIDEO GAMES, and other forms of inactivity
are replaced with appropriate EXERCISE, and get people moving.

Success will come:
When we love our bodies as much as our cars.

"Choosing to make America healthier"

By Michael Milken
San Diego Union-Tribune
June 13, 2008

San Diego's thousands of biotechnology researchers work in a field of mind-boggling complexity that requires years of rigorous training. They can tell you how hard it is to make even small advances against major diseases.

So assuming you don't have an advanced scientific degree, you might think there's nothing you can do to achieve the kind of medical breakthroughs that would eliminate half the diabetes cases prevent one of every five cancer deaths, and save trillions of dollars. Anyone who developed a pill that could do that would win a Nobel Prize.

You have that pill. It's called lifestyle choice. And it's free.

The fact that lifestyle affects health isn't news. But in a recent report, the Milken Institute showed lifestyle's economic impact – how our choices contribute to chronic diseases that increase treatment and insurance costs, reduce productivity, erode our international competitiveness and, worst of all, magnify personal suffering.

The report, "An Unhealthy America: The Economic Burden of Chronic Disease," quantifies the staggering costs of "failing to contain the containable." In this presidential election year, we need more focus on these costs, which undermine prospects for extending health insurance coverage and for coping with the medical burden of an aging population. The opportunity costs also include diversion of skilled research and clinical talent to chronic-disease care.

For every dollar we spend on treatment, we lose three to four times as much indirectly. When chronically ill workers take sick days, their absenteeism reduces the supply of labor and with it the gross domestic product. But the greatest GDP impact is from "presenteeism," which reduces output when sick employees show up for work to avoid losing wages and then perform below par. Combining the diversion of caregivers with the costs of absenteeism and presenteeism, the total impact of chronic disease already exceeds $1 trillion a year, including more than $100 billion in California alone.

This cost is one of three interdependent health policy concerns. The second is the cost of advanced research. Third is the system of distributing and paying for medical services so all Americans have access to high-quality care. If we address all three with good policy decisions, we can assure longer life spans and higher quality of life at substantially reduced cost.

But we need to start now. By mid-century, the preventable impact of seven chronic diseases – diabetes, pulmonary conditions, hypertension, mental disorders, heart disease, cancers and stroke – could reduce annual GDP by six trillion dollars a year.

Behavioral choices – especially those that underlie obesity – often affect the prevalence, severity and costs of these diseases. While genetic factors are very important, as much as 70 percent of direct health care spending is to treat lifestyle-related conditions. In calculating cost savings, our report assumed only a modest reduction in the percentage of overweight and obese Americans from the current two-thirds to about half.

We can and should do better. One of every four Americans is now more than 20 percent above ideal body weight, the dividing line between overweight and obese. That's up from one in eight as recently as 1990. What if we turned the clock back only a decade, returning to 1998 obesity levels? The impact would be 15 million fewer cases of the seven chronic diseases by 2023. In that year alone, without adjusting for inflation, we would reduce health care spending by $60 billion and increase productivity by $254 billion. In fact, the single most effective way to reduce the burden of disease and lower costs is to reduce obesity.

No one claims it's easy to change diet and exercise habits. In my case, it took a doctor saying, "You have cancer." Yet we've made progress against smoking – another entrenched habit – and I believe we can do the same with obesity.

It's also vital that we build on our national commitment to medical research. If we continue cutting back on research, we risk losing a generation of young physician-scientists. Unfortunately, recent National Institutes of Health budgets have declined in real terms. That trend has a large impact on San Diego because of this area's many life-sciences laboratories. Yet with better cooperation among industry, academic and government researchers, we can still make real progress toward life-saving cures. If that means eliminating some bureaucratic regulations that limit joint public-private efforts, let's do it.

America woke up 50 years ago when Sputnik shocked us into action. We need similar resolve today so chronic diseases don't undermine our economy from within the way the Soviet challenge of the 1950s threatened our security from without. Each of us can help by taking reasonable steps to reduce our personal chronic-disease risks. Progress against the preventable cost of these diseases will free up the human, social and financial capital we need to fund crucial research and provide high-quality healthcare to all Americans.

* * * * * * * * * * * * * * * * * *

The Immune System

Adenoide

Tonsils

mph Nodes

Thymus

umphatic
Vessels

Spleen

peyer's
Patches

ppendix

Bone
Marrow

he human immune system must protect every
uare inch of the body, both inside and out.

addition to specific organs, the immune system
cludes billions of warrior cells that patrol the
ntire body, on the lookout for any signs of trouble.

Our Immune System

*What we know about it ...
and what we don't.*

This is the system that protects us from being invaded by troublesome viruses. This is our private army of warriors that fight any enemy that would cause trouble in our body.

These soldiers need the required weapons to fight these invaders and they get it through the food we eat — and with the right diet. They do their job — superbly.

The main secret of success is top level nutrition, as well as other common lifestyle programs, like exercise.

This then, is the main requirement for good health. The trillions of cells in antibodies need to be fed nutritious food only. Any harmful food will break down its functions, and result in disease.

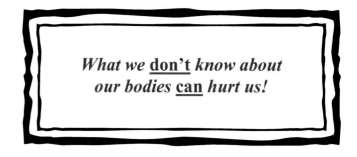

*What we __don't__ know about
our bodies __can__ hurt us!*

There are several other systems in our bodies; one in particular is the repair system. A good example is when we get a cut there is an immediate response and all forces go to work and focus on the area of the damage. These forces respond with the necessary materials and know how to do the repair, depending on the extent of damage and other factors. Like hygiene, age, conditions, etc., the repair is done in the shortest possible time — it is the <u>ONLY VALID</u> healing procedure that works.

It is best not to interfere with this natural process by trying to speed things up. We just need to use good hygiene and let nature do the rest.

This repair crew does more than heal cuts — it is on 24-hour care-giving missions, and is at work even when we sleep. Let's make sure we give it the tools it needs to do its job — **that is a good healthy diet.**

The main secret of success is top level nutrition, as well as other common lifestyle programs, like exercise.

"Fast facts"

(Editor's note: How to go on a fast without hurting yourself!)

R.J. Ignelzi
San Diego Union-Tribune
June 24, 2008

Although short-term fasting may offer some benefits, it also comes with risks. If you're determined to fast, for whatever reasons, consider these precautions.

Fast for short periods of time only. Going without food for one or two days is usually OK as long as you have adequate hydration and no health problems.

Hydrate with lots of drinks containing sodium and electrolytes, such as Pedialyte.

At the end of the fast, slowly introduce nutritious foods, avoiding bingeing and junk food. When fasting, be careful driving or operating machinery since you might feel lightheaded. If you have lots of weight to lose and are determined to fast longer than three days, consult your doctor first. A medically supervised, modified fast may be suggested.

Certain people should not fast, including those with diabetes, women who are pregnant or nursing, children, elderly, anyone with an irregular heartbeat and people taking prescription medications, which can be toxic to the kidneys during a fast.

Anyone who has or has had an eating disorder should steer clear of fasts.

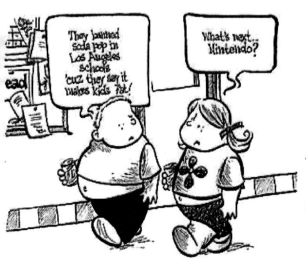

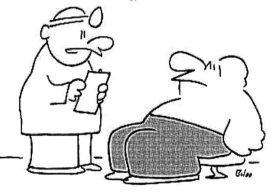

"LET'S EASE INTO THIS--I WANT YOU TO TRY FASTING BETWEEN MEALS."

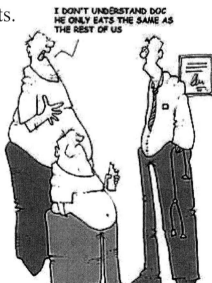

3

"Portion, serving sizes are different"

By Nina Marinello
New York Times News Service/*San Diego Union-Tribune*
June 24, 2008

QUESTION: Does "serving size" and "portion size" mean the same thing?

ANSWER: Although these terms are often used together, they mean different things when it comes to our diet.

A "serving" is the recommended amount of food nutrition that experts advise us to eat. Serving sizes keep calories, fat and sugar in check. Serving sizes are listed on the Nutrition Facts label or food packages.

However, how much of a particular food we choose to eat is the "portion." For example, a cup o brown rice (equal to two servings) and a large apple (also equal to two servings) are realistic portions and a good source of nutrients. But a 2-cup portion of ice cream (four 1/2-cup servings) has more calories, fat and sugar than is recommended on a daily basis.

Consuming larger portions is expected every now and then, but indulging too often can lead us down a slippery slope called "portion distortion." The general consensus is that the increase in calories consumed because of larger portions has contributed to the obesity epidemic Unfortunately, most of us have lost sight of what a normal portion looks like.

This is partly because competition for customers led fast-food restaurants to offer "super-sized" meals. The appeal of larger portions also created mega-sized candy bars, monstrous muffins and jugs of soda.

Did you know that over the past 20 years, a typical bagel has grown from 3 inches to 6 inches in diameter? How about muffins, which have increased almost five times their original size?
Expecting large portions away from home has created a habit of serving ourselves larger portions at the kitchen table. Adding to the problem is the fact that even our dinner plates are larger than they were 20 years ago. We still tend to fill them up. Short of getting Grandma's dishes out of the attic, what can you do?

MEAL Portions Today Compared to 20 years ago

At restaurants you can share meals, order smaller portions if available, bring half home or eat ss on the days when you will be going out to eat to save room for the extra calories. At home, e measured serving utensils, control second helpings and avoid eating out of cookie boxes and ip bags.

Get into the habit of reading the nutrition labels and become more aware of recommended rving sizes. To find out how many servings would be a healthy portion for you, consult a etitian, pick up a nutrition book like "The American Dietetic Association Complete Food and utrition Guide" or go online to eatright.org.

Although many of us have good intentions when choosing serving sizes, it's still difficult to). To help you, The National Heart Lung and Blood Institute provides a handy serving-size iide. It uses common items to visually keep servings in check. For example, half of a baseball ould equal "cup of pasta, rice, fresh fruit or ice cream," which all equal one serving. Three nces of meat, poultry or fish equals a deck of cards. A compact disc is about the size of one ncake serving.

To help with portion control, buy three-sectioned picnic plates. Fill the largest section with getables or salad, and the smaller sections each with a starch like pasta, potato or rice, and a otein like meat, fish, poultry or tofu. As long as you don't pile too high, this approach can help ou achieve better portion control.

TODAY 2008

20 YEARS AGO

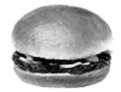

333 CALORIES

8000 Calories

Nutrition Fact Labels

Serving Size
This tells you what is considered one (1) serving of the product. Every other nutrient listed on the label is based on this amount.

Calories
Calories are a unit of energy. Calories in food come from carbohydrate, protein and fat. Because calories give us energy, we need them to be able to think and be active.

% Daily Value
This tells you the percentage of the daily value you are getting, which is the recommended amount of a nutrient you need per day. A food that has more than 20% of the Daily Value of a certain nutrient is a good source of that nutrient.

Cholesterol
Cholesterol is only found in animal products. You should avoid eating too much cholesterol, especially if your blood is high in cholesterol.

Total Carbohydrate
Carbohydrates give your muscles and brain energy. Certain types of carbohydrates are sometimes listed on the label:

Fiber: This helps with digestion and keeps you full between meals.

Sugars: These are important for instant energy, but eating too much can be unhealthy.

Nutrition Facts
Serving Size
Servings per Container

Amount Per Serving

Calories   Calories from Fat

% Daily Value*

Total Fat
  Saturated Fat
  Trans Fat
  Polyunsaturated Fat
  Monounsaturated Fat
Cholesterol
Sodium
Total Carbohydrate
  Dietary Fiber
  Sugars
  Other Carb.
Protein

Vitamin A	Vitamin C
Calcium	Iron

* Percent Daily Values are based on a 2,000 -calorie diet. Your daily values may be higher or lower depending on your calorie needs:

	Calories	2,000	2,500
Total Fat	Less than	65 g	80 g
Sat. Fat	Less than	20 g	25 g
Cholesterol	Less than	300 mg	300 mg
Sodium	Less than	2,400 mg	2,400 mg
Total Carbohydrate		300 g	375 g
Dietary Fiber		25 g	30 g

Calories per gram:
  Fat 9   Carbohydrate 4   Protein 4

AMERICAN MEASURING SYSTEM IS MORE DESIREABLE AND UNDERSTANDABLE, WE NEED TO CHANGE OUR NUTRITION FACT LABEL LAWS IN ORDER TO UNDERSTAND WHAT WE ARE EATING.   A GOOD EXAMPLE IS:
4 GRAMS = 1 TEASPOON OF SUGAR
40 GRAMS = 10 TEASPOONS OF SUGAR
THIS IS WHAT SHOULD BE STATED ON THE LABEL.

Footnote
This reminds us that all of the Daily Values come from the recommendations for a 2,000-calorie meal plan. Most adolescents need more than this amount as they grow in height, build muscles, and stay active. Your needs may be higher or lower; keep in mind this is just an average. These Daily Value percentages (%) are not for everyone.

Servings Per Container
This tells you how many servings you can get from one package. Some containers are a single serving, but most have more than one serving per package.

Calories from Fat
This is the number of calories that come from fat. It is not the percent of fat in the food.

Total Fat
Fat is essential in our bodies. There are 4 kinds of fat. Monounsaturated and polyunsaturated fat are the kinds of fat that are healthy for heart. Saturated fat and trans fat are not heart healthy and should be limited.

Sodium
Sodium tells you how much salt is in the food. People with high blood pressure are sometimes told to follow a low sodium diet. Eating less than 2400 mg of sodium every day is recommended.

Protein
This nutrient is used to build muscle and fight infections. Teen girls usually need around 60 grams of protein each day.

Vitamins/Minerals
This section tells you the percent daily value for Vitamin A, Vitamin C, Calcium, and Iron you are getting from this product. Other vitamins and minerals may be included in this section.

This bar of candy has 84 grams of **SUGAR** = 22 teaspoons
Did you know that?!

But you can't tell that from the wrapper unless you know how to read it.
Here's the "real" formula: Only one-fourth of this candy bar = a whopping 21 grams of sugar.
Multiply that by four to learn that this one candy bar contains 84 grams of sugar = 22 teaspoons!

* 4 grams of sugar = 1 tsp., so 84 grams ÷ 4 = 22 tsp.

Nutrition Facts

Serving Size 1/4 bar (35 g)
Servings Per Container 4

Calories 170
Calories from Fat 90

Amount Per Serving	% Daily Value*
Total Fat 10 g	**15%**
Saturated Fat 6 g	**29%**
Trans Fat 0 g	
Cholesterol < 5 mg	**1%**
Sodium 15 mg	**1%**
Vitamin A 0% • Vitamin C 0%	

Amount Per Serving	% Daily Value*
Total Carbohydrate 23 g	**8%**
Dietary Fiber <1 g	**3%**
Sugars 21 g	
Protein 1 g	
• Calcium 4% • Iron 0%	

*Percent Daily Values are based on a 2,000 calorie diet. Your daily values may be higher or lower depending on your calorie needs:

	Calories	2,000	2,500
Total Fat	Less than	65 g	80 g
Sat Fat	Less than	20 g	25 g
Cholesterol	Less than	300 mg	300 mg
Sodium	Less than	2,400 mg	2,400 mg
Total Carbohydrate		300 g	375 g
Dietary Fiber		25 g	30 g

INGREDIENTS: MILK CHOCOLATE (SUGAR, CHOCOLATE, COCOA BUTTER, NONFAT MILK, MILKFAT, LACTOSE, SOY LECITHIN, PGPR – AN EMULSIFIER, VANILLIN – AN ARTIFICIAL FLAVOR). MADE ON EQUIPMENT THAT ALSO PROCESSES PEANUTS AND NUTS.

DISTRIBUTED BY NESTLÉ USA, INC., GLENDALE, CA 91203 USA
MADE IN BRAZIL BY NESTLÉ BRAZIL, Ltda. Nestleusa.com Ⓤ D 455385-2

Questions or Comments?
Call 1-800-258-6728, M-F, 8AM-8PM ET.
Visit us any time at NestleClassics.com

NESTLÉ is a registered trademark of Société des Produits Nestlé S.A., Vevey, Switzerland.

0 28000 15220 8

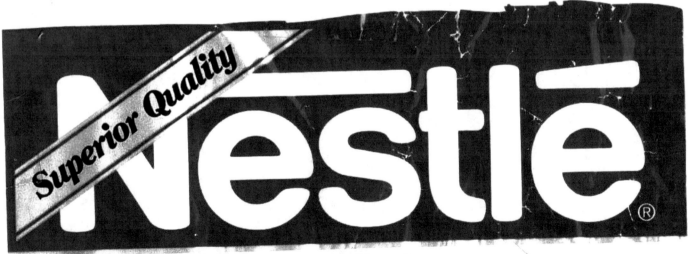

Superior Quality

Nestlé®
Milk Chocolate

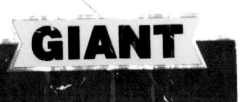
GIANT

NET WT 5 OZ (141.7 g)

What Are You Drinking?

Soda cans are 12 fluid oz

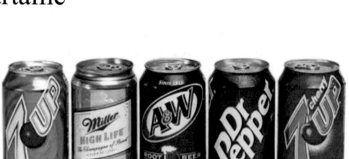

Manufacturers list nutritional values as:

Coca Cola Zero	58mg	Aspartame
Coca Cola Classic	39g	Sugar
Diet Coke	125mg	Aspartame
Fanta Orange	35g	Sugar
Fanta Strawberry	33g	Sugar
Fanta Grape	35g	Sugar

12 fl. Oz. can = 52g = 16 tsp. of sugar per can = 122 calories

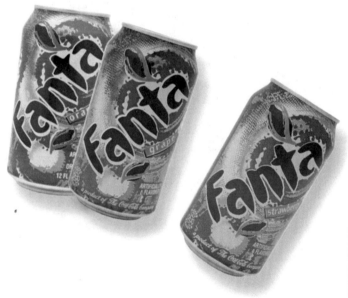

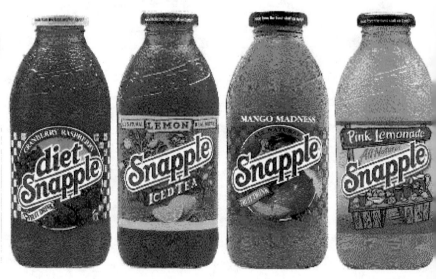

Diet Drinks - Aspartame

(Author: aspartame is an additive commonly used to sweeten "sugar free" beverages.)

Dr. Betty Martini, D. Hum
Source: www.rense.com
July 5, 2008

It's not the caffeine, it's the aspartame. It has free methyl alcohol which is classified as a narcotic. It causes chronic methanol poisoning, which affects the dopamine system of the brain and causes the addiction. Here is Dr. H. J. Roberts' report on the addiction published in Townsend Letter for Doctors: www.dorway.com/tldaddic.html

ASPARTAME MAKES YOU FATTER!
Here's how aspartame makes you gain weight:

Position Statement from Dr. Sandra Cabot
Mission Possible Australia **(excerpted)**
www.liverdoctor.com

I have been a medical doctor for over 25 years and have clinical and research interests in the liver and metabolism. I have authored several best selling health books including the "Liver Cleansing Diet," "The Body Shaping Diet," "Don't Let Your Hormones Ruin Your Life," "Women's Health," "Menopause and Natural Hormone Replacement Therapy," and I lecture internationally on these subjects. I have been consulted by thousands of patients with weight problems, hormonal imbalances, fatty liver, sluggish metabolism and chronic ill health. I have been an advocate and practitioner of nutritional methods of healing for 30 years. I regularly appear on national television and broadcast on many radio stations to educate people about the importance of a healthy liver in achieving good health and weight control!

In the interests of public health I am making a position statement concerning the use of the artificial sweetener called aspartame and sold most commonly under the names of NutraSweet and Equal. One must ask, "Why do millions of people ingest a toxic chemical like aspartame everyday"? To me it appears ridiculous and I believe that it is because people have been brainwashed into thinking aspartame will keep their weight down and is good for health. It also shows me that we have lost touch with our own natural senses and instincts.

4

After having been consulted by thousands of overweight people suffering with problem concerning the liver and/or metabolism I can assure you that aspartame will not help you in any way, indeed it will help you to gain unwanted weight. This has been my experience, and there are logical reasons to explain the fattening and bloating effects of aspartame.

When you ingest the toxic chemical aspartame it is absorbed from the intestines and passes immediately to the LIVER where it is taken inside the liver via the liver filter. The liver then breaks down or metabolizes aspartame to its toxic components — phenylalanine, aspartic acid and methanol. This process requires a lot of energy from the liver, which means there will be less energy remaining in the liver cells. This means the liver cells will have less energy for fa burning and metabolism, which will result in fat storing. Excess fat may build up inside the liver cells causing "fatty liver" and when this starts to occur it is extremely difficult to lose weight. In my vast experience any time that you overload the liver you will increase the tendency to gain weight easily.

Aspartame also causes weight gain by other mechanisms — Causes unstable blood sugar levels. which increases the appetite and causes cravings for sweets/sugar. Thus it is particularly toxic for those with diabetes or epilepsy. Causes fluid retention giving the body a puffy and bloated appearance. This makes people look fatter than they are and increases cellulite.

Aspartame (NutraSweet/Equal/Spoonful/Canderel/E951/Benevia) is an addictive excitoneurotoxic carcinogenic drug that interacts with virtually all drugs and vaccines. Here are the references:

Aspartame Disease: "An Ignored Epidemic," www.sunsentpress.com by H. J. Roberts, M.D. , 1000-page medical text on this plague.

Dying for a Diet Coke: www.rense.com/general78/dying.htm

Aspartame Information List: www.mpwhi.com scroll down to banners
These athletes using aspartame are an accident about to happen (or anyone for that matter): www.mpwhi.com/george_carlin_and_diet_coke.htm

* * * * * * * * * * * * * * * * * * *

Energy Drinks

Do you know that 3 1/2 cans of RED BULL are as potent as one can (8.4 oz) of Spike Shooter?

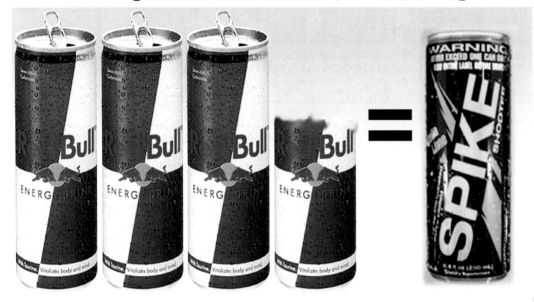

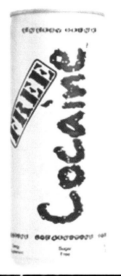

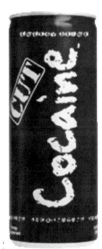

RECOMMENDED USE: Begin use with one-half can daily to determine tolerance. Never exceed one can daily.

CAUTION: This product contains strong stimulants and should not be combined with any other stimulant or fat-loss product.

WARNING: DO NOT USE IF YOU ARE UNDER THE AGE OF 18 OR ELDERLY. NOT TAKE WITH ANY OTHER STIMULANT OR WEIGHT-LOSS SUPPLEMENT ANY PRESCRIPTION OR OVER-THE-COUNTER MEDICINE. Do not use if you pregnant or nursing or at risk of being treated for high-blood pressure, heart ease, hyperthyroidism, spasms, psychiatric disease, suffer from migraines, e asthma, or are taking asthma medication. Discontinue use if you experience ziness, headache, nausea, or heart palpitations. If you have trouble sleeping. not take within 6 hours of bedtime. KEEP OUT OF REACH OF CHILDREN.

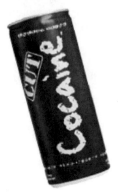
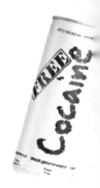

Caffeine Buddies Up to Cocaine

With friends like this, who needs enemies?

Do you know that one can (8.4 oz) of Cocaine has 4 1/2 teaspoons of sugar and 280mg of Caffeine per 8oz?

*Cocaine (available again in the U.S.) is a highly caffeinated energy drink distributed by Redux Beverages. It contains 350% as much caffeine as the most-popular energy drink, Red Bull, symbolized by three and a half steer heads on the label. Aside from caffeine the label boasts 750 milligrams of taurine, another common ingredient found in many energy drinks.

Cocaine was pulled from U.S. shelves as a result of the FDA's decision that Cocaine was "illegally marketing their drink as an alternative to street drugs". Redux Beverages began working on a new name for the product immediately. At the end of May, 2007, the Redux team decided to change the name to "No Name:" energy drink, with the new can label (sometimes still with the original can just covered by a plastic sleeve with the new name, allowing it to be peeled off revealing the old one) featuring a large blank space for fans to write their chosen name for the drink, covering the "Cocaine" on the can itself. On 17 June 2007, the drink was redistributed in the U.S. under the new labeling.

However, Redux Beverages has recently announced that the drink will return to shelves under its original name in early 2008[1]. Cocaine's founder and senior partner, Jamey Kirby, always believed they would get their name back. Said Kirby in June 2007, "Oh, we'll get our name back. We'll get it back." And they did. Cocaine is now being sold as "Cocaine" and can be found on the shelves of many stores around the U.S.[2]

The drink is available online or in local beverage stores around the U.S. The beverage is also available in Europe, where it has always been sold as Cocaine Energy Drink rather than Insert Name Here: (as it was briefly sold in the U.S).

This article is quoted from Wikipedia.org and can be read in its entirety at
http://en.wikipedia.org/wiki/Cocaine_%28drink%29.

Healthy Drinks?

s this a good health food for sick people?

**This drink contains 22g of sugar
which = 5 1/2 teaspoons of sugar**

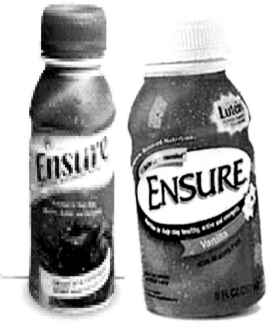

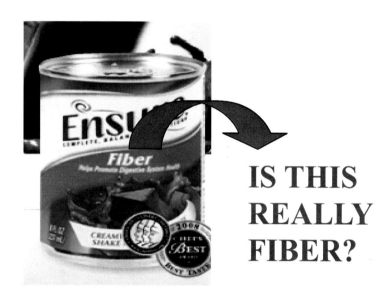

**IS THIS
REALLY
FIBER?**

The question is do you want all this OIL and SUGAR in your body?

| VITAMINS AND MINERALS | NUTRITION FACTS | INGREDIENTS |

(U)D WATER, CORN MALTODEXTRIN, SUGAR (SUCROSE), MILK PROTEIN CONCENTRATE, CANOLA OIL, SOY PROTEIN CONCENTRATE, CORN OIL, COCOA POWDER (PROCESSED WITH ALKALI), SHORT-CHAIN FRUCTOOLIGOSACCHARIDES, WHEY PROTEIN CONCENTRATE, NATURAL AND ARTIFICIAL FLAVORS, SOY LECITHIN, CARRAGEENAN, POTASSIUM CITRATE, MAGNESIUM PHOSPHATE, SODIUM CITR/ ⊃ More

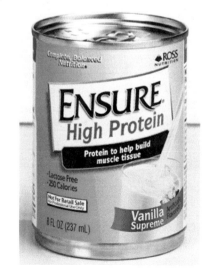

Is putting this much SUGAR in your body healthy?
34g of sugars = 8 1/2 teaspoons of sugar

What about the FAT and OILS and HARMFUL chemicals

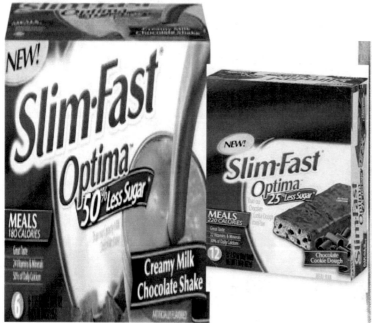

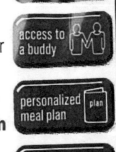

for **FREE** weight loss support and tools to customize your weight loss journey, go to **Slim-Fast.com** or call **1-800-SLIMFAST**

advice & support

access to a buddy

personalized meal plan

registered dietitian

weight on with one Slim•Fast Meal a day, your sensible eating habits and daily physical activity. Return to the weight loss plan if you start regaining the weight.

If you want to lose weight & are under 18, pregnant, nursing, following a diet recommended by a doctor, have health problems such as diabetes, or want to lose more than 30 lbs., see a doctor before starting this or any diet. Do not lose more than 2 pounds a week after the first week. Rapid weight loss may cause health problems. Do not use as a sole source of nutrition. Eat at least 1,200 calories a day.

Nutrition Facts

Serving Size 1 Can (325.0 g)

Amount Per Serving	
Calories 220	Calories from Fat 27
	% Daily Value*
Total Fat 3.0g	5%
Saturated Fat 1.0g	5%
Polyunsaturated Fat 0.5g	
Monounsaturated Fat 1.5g	
Cholesterol 5mg	2%
Sodium 220mg	9%
Total Carbohydrates 40.0g	13%
Dietary Fiber 5.0g	20%
Sugars 34.0g	
Protein 10.0g	
Vitamin A 3% •	Vitamin C 100%
Calcium 40% •	Iron 15%

* Based on a 2000 calorie diet

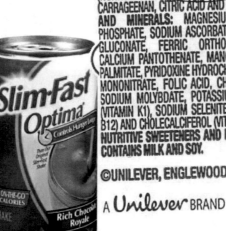

INGREDIENTS: FAT FREE MILK, WATER, SUGAR, COCOA (PROCESSED WITH ALKALI), CANOLA OIL, FRUCTOSE, CALCIUM CASEINATE, GUM ARABIC, CELLULOSE GEL, HYDROGENATED SOYBEAN OIL, MONO AND DIGLYCERIDES, POTASSIUM PHOSPHATE, SOYBEAN LECITHIN, CELLULOSE GUM, CARRAGEENAN, ISOLATED SOY PROTEIN, ARTIFICIAL FLAVOR, MALTODEXTRIN, SUCRALOSE AND ACESULFAME POTASSIUM (NONNUTRITIVE SWEETENERS), DEXTROSE, POTASSIUM CARRAGEENAN, CITRIC ACID AND SODIUM CITRATE. VITAMINS AND MINERALS: MAGNESIUM PHOSPHATE, CALCIUM PHOSPHATE, SODIUM ASCORBATE, VITAMI GLUCONATE, FERRIC ORTHOPHOSPHA CALCIUM PANTOTHENATE, MANGANESE S PALMITATE, PYRIDOXINE HYDROCHLORIDE, F MONONITRATE, FOLIC ACID, CHROMIUM SODIUM MOLYBDATE, POTASSIUM IODID (VITAMIN K1), SODIUM SELENITE, CYANOC B12) AND CHOLECALCIFEROL (VITAMIN D3) NUTRITIVE SWEETENERS AND NONNUTR CONTAINS MILK AND SOY.

©UNILEVER, ENGLEWOOD CLIFFS

A *Unilever* BRAND

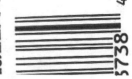

These are only few ingredients in Slim Fast that we are aware of. Could you even imagine all the harmful chemical and additives that are added to this drink which we are not aware of?

"Steering teens away from drugs, alcohol"

By Sharon Heilbrunn
San Diego Union-Tribune
June 7, 2008

As a 30-year officer with the San Diego Police Department working vice, drugs and narcotics, Phillip Hubbs has seen it all.

Prostitution. Teen murders. Children who know more about methamphetamine than most adults.

Fifteen years ago, Hubbs watched as the San Diego department eliminated the Drug and Resistance Education (DARE) program because of budget cuts. Motivated by the ugliness he had seen in his line of work, Hubbs founded the nonprofit PRONASA, or Proactive Network Against Substance Abuse, five years ago. Along with a team of mostly law enforcement officers, he now delivers presentations to middle and high school students throughout the region about the consequences of drug use. "We need kids to understand the dangers and consequences of their actions," Hubbs said.

Hubbs takes his program a step further than DARE, which focuses mostly on teaching elementary school children to "Just Say No." He saw the need for educating not only middle and high school students, but also parents, nurses, coaches and teachers.

"We've evolved from DARE," Hubbs said. "We began our program in East County, and it exploded, and now it's everywhere from Chula Vista to Oceanside." With the recent drug raids involving San Diego State University students, where dozens were arrested in connection with a variety of narcotics charges, Hubbs knows it's more relevant than ever to help vulnerable teenagers.

> *"We need kids to understand the dangers and \consequences of their actions," Hubbs said.*

"The accessibility of drugs and the evolution of technology, like cell phones and the Internet, i the biggest problem," Hubbs said. "With technology, kids are always going to be several step ahead of law enforcement."

So he makes sure PRONASA's message is consistent. He doesn't speak down to students. H knows they are resourceful. But he also knows they think they are invincible. And then there mom and dad. "Parents are always in denial that their children are involved," Hubbs said. "W want to give parents tools for communication, what to look for, and also resources."

Hubbs, still an active detective, puts at least 12 to 18 hours a week into PRONASA. Annually the organization delivers more than 50 presentations to students and adults throughout th county. Hubbs, an Alpine resident, said about half are in East County communities.

Hubbs gave three assemblies to students at Valhalla High School in El Cajon on May 16, th day before the school's prom. When he speaks, there's no song and dance. McGruff the dog isn there to "take a bite out of crime." He doesn't preach. Hubbs speaks firsthand about what h knows.

In Valhalla's theater, 150 students listened intently as Hubbs showed images of haggar methamphetamine users and teenagers being wheeled away on gurneys after drinking too muc in Tijuana. **He talked about the dangers of ingesting prescription drugs o energy drinks,** or inhaling aerosol fumes.

But what really hit home were his examples – some shown through the news, others tol firsthand – of students from nearby schools who had died from drug overdoses or drunker driving casualties. Cheerleaders. Varsity football players. People their age.

"I have a very strong message," Hubbs said. "I'm able to show news segments on kids who hav died. It makes direct contact with students. Sometimes they know the student, or the school."

Brooke Wilson, a senior, has heard friends making plans to drink the night of prom.
"This presentation was insightful," she said. "It's a good reminder."

* * * * * * * * *

'Binge drinking proves deadly for more college-age victims"

(Author: Like sugar, alcohol is addictive and detrimental to your health.)

By Amy Forliti
Associated Press/*San Diego Union-Tribune*
July 8, 2008

WINONA, MINN. — On the morning after the house party on Johnson Street, Jenna Foellmi and several other twenty-somethings lay sprawled on beds and couches. When a friend reached over to wake her, Foellmi was cold to the touch.

The friend's screams woke up the others still asleep in the house. Foellmi, 20, a biochemistry major at Winona State University, died of alcohol poisoning Dec. 14, one day after she had finished her last exam of the semester. According to police reports, she had three beers during the day, then played beer pong — a drinking game — in the evening, and downed some vodka, too.

Foellmi's death was tragic, but typical in many ways.

An Associated Press analysis of federal records found that 157 college-age people, between the ages of 18 and 23, drank themselves to death from 1999 through 2005, the most recent year for which figures are available. The number of alcohol-poisoning deaths per year nearly doubled over that span, from 18 in 1999 to a peak of 35 in 2005, though the total went up and down from year to year and dipped as low as 14 in 2001.

"There have always been problems with young people and alcohol, but it just seems like they are a little more intense now than they used to be," said Connie Gores, vice president for student life at Winona State. "The goal of a lot of them is just to get smashed."

Over the seven-year span, 83 of the college-age victims were, like Foellmi, under the legal drinking age of 21.

A separate AP analysis of hundreds of news articles about alcohol-poisoning deaths in the past decade found that victims drank themselves well past the point of oblivion — with an average blood-alcohol level of 0.4 percent, or five times the legal limit for driving.

Schools and communities have responded in a variety of ways, including programs to teach incoming freshmen about the dangers of extreme drinking, designating professors to help students avoid overdoing it, and passing laws to discourage binge drinking.

5

Some universities are trying to send a message with Web sites and programs that feature slogan such as "Remember Last Night."

San Diego State University has a Web site that lets students punch in information about thei drinking habits and learn about the risks. Winona State is starting an online course to teach incoming freshmen the dangers of excessive drinking.

Forty professors at California State University Fresno have taken a pledge to learn about the effects of alcohol misuse and to advise students. The professors' names are on posters aroun campus. Other universities have banned or restricted alcohol advertising and sponsorships i athletics.

* * * * * * * * * * * * * * * * * * * *

Binge drinking can liquidate your life.

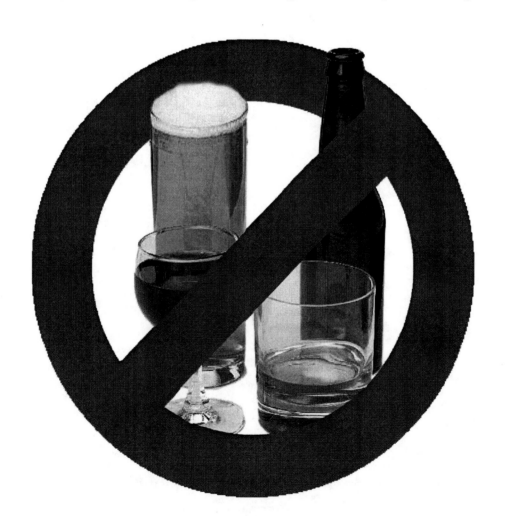

FOOD ADDITIVES

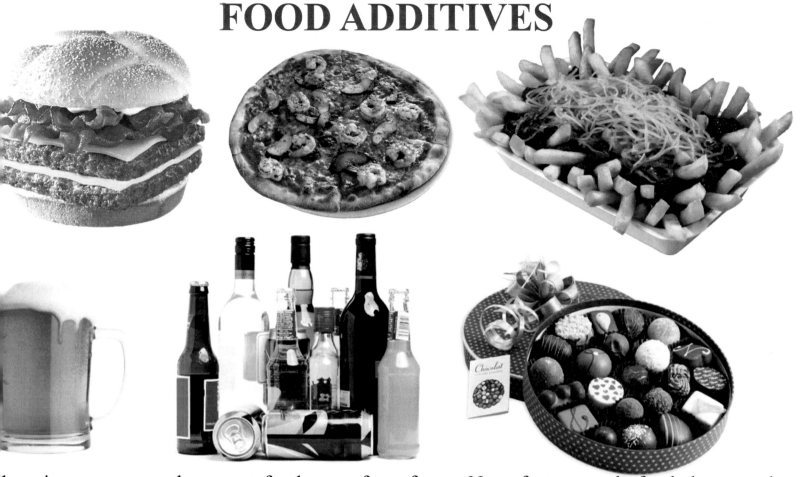

hopping was easy when most food came from farms. Now, factory-made foods have made hemical additives a significant part of our diet. Most people may not be able to pronounce the ames of many of these chemicals, but they still want to know what the chemicals do, which nes are safe and which are poorly tested, or possibly dangerous.

> *A simple general rule about additives is to avoid sodium nitrite, saccharin, caffeine, olestra, acesulfame K, and artificial coloring. Not only are they among the most questionable additives, but they are used primarily in foods of low nutritional value.*

lso, don't forget the two most familiar additives: **sugar and salt**. They may pose the reatest risk because we consume so much of them. Fortunately, most additives are safe and ome even increase the nutritional value of the food.

"Supplement called 'fountain of youth'"

By Cheryl Clark, Staff Writer
San Diego Union-Tribune
June 16, 2008

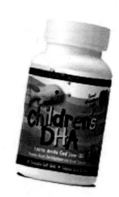

San Diego – Healthy seniors who take DHEA tablets to protect memory or pep up their sex live are wasting money, according to a yearlong UCSD study that found no gains from the over-the counter hormone supplement.

"This product is touted everywhere like it's the fountain of youth," said Donna Kritz-Silverstei at the UCSD School of Medicine and lead author of the report.

"But when we looked (at) . . . cognitive function, mood, sexual function and feelings of genera well-being, it didn't seem to provide any benefit," said Kritz-Silverstein, whose study wa published in the May issue of the *Journal of the American Geriatrics Society*. The Nationa Institute on Aging funded the research.
The body's adrenal glands make DHEA, or dehydroepiandrosterone, out of cholesterol. DHEA i then converted into two important hormones – testosterone and estrogen.

DHEA production declines gradually during life, starting when people are in their mid-20s. B the time individuals reach 70, their DHEA levels are about one-fifth of the peak. Consume interest in DHEA supplements took off in the 1990s, and U.S. sales of the product totaled abou $55 million last year. It costs nearly $100 for a year's supply of pills that amount to 50 mg a day the amount required to achieve peak levels of DHEA in the bloodstream.

Studies on the effects of DHEA have been limited, and their findings have been mixed.

"There is little scientific evidence to support the use of DHEA as a 'rejuvenating' hormone," th National Institute on Aging said on its Web site.

The agency also said early signs suggest that DHEA supplements **might cause problems suc as liver damage and raise the risk of breast and prostate cancer** by adversely influencin levels of testosterone and estrogen.

n the 1990s, some studies found that mice and rats showed greater learning and memory apacity after receiving doses of DHEA. "That prompted some people to speculate that if you ould restore DHEA levels to that of youth, perhaps you could improve health overall," Kritz-ilverstein said. In recent years, certain studies recorded no benefits from DHEA supplements.

)thers suggested that people who receive boosts of DHEA have improved libido and memory kills. But Kritz-Silverstein said those studies weren't definitive because they tested DHEA upplements for only a few weeks or months, enrolled very small numbers of participants and idn't focus on people old enough to start suffering age-related cognitive impairment. "So the nly way to determine whether they have any benefits is to conduct good, scientific, placebo-ontrolled clinical trials to see if they work," she said. The University of California San Diego tudy enrolled 225 healthy men and women in the San Diego area ages 55 to 85. Half of them ook 50 mg of DHEA pills per day, while the other half took placebo pills.

'articipants were examined for depression, perceptions of physical and emotional health, atisfaction with life and sexual function throughout the study. When the results were tallied, We really didn't see any change over the year between those who were taking DHEA and those vho were not," Kritz-Silverstein said.

)r. Thomas Perls, a specialist in the anti-aging industry at the Boston University School of Medicine, said claims that DHEA supplements rejuvenate healthy seniors are a "sign of **nedical quackery.**"

Vhile there might be limited benefit in giving DHEA supplements to younger people with onditions that cause abnormally low DHEA levels, he said, "I'm not familiar with any studies howing a beneficial effect on young or old individuals aging normally"

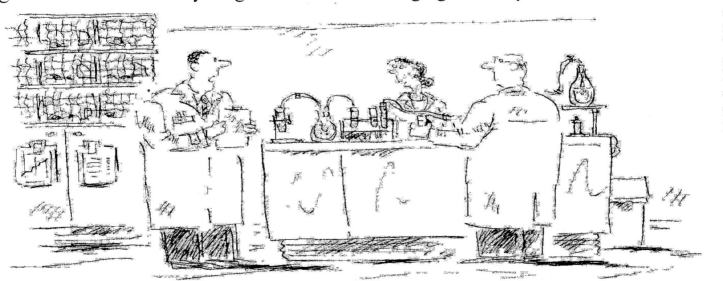

"It's fine to discover cures, but , remember,
chronic conditions are our bread and butter."

"Analysts see business of candy as 'recession-proof'

Consumers willing to pay for sweets"

By Martha Irvine
Associated Press/ *San Diego Union-Tribune*
June 30, 2008

CHICAGO — Like a lot of people, Nate Towne is cutting back on spending. He's carpooling t work and only shops at grocery stores that take coupons or offer discount "rewards" cards. But even in this economy, he remains a self-described "candy snob."

"I'm serious when I say I'll pay a premium for my top favorites because in the grand scheme o things, it's only a few bucks," said Towne, a 37-year-old public relations consultant in Madison Wis.

He's not the only one who's stuck on candy. **Americans buy billions of dollars worth of th stuff each year** – with more than $29 billion in retail sales in 2007, according to the Nationa Confectioners Association. That's about a 3 percent increase from the previous year.

That sizable sweet tooth is a big reason many analysts say the **candy business is likely to far better than other nonessentials in these economically trying times**, even as prices fo commodities such as sugar, milk and cocoa have risen. The bottom line is: As vices go, candy i still relatively cheap for most consumers.

"People may not be able to flip for Starbucks or even to go to McDonald's. But they have th ability to pay a dollar for a treat," said Jim Tillotson, professor of food policy and internationa business at Tufts University's Fletcher School.

Analysts at The Nielsen Co., which tracks consumer habits, go as far as calling the **candy business "recession-proof,"** compared with other discretionary items, such as tobacco anc carbonated beverages (though beer also tends to do well when the economy is hurting).

They note that consumers are cutting back on longer-distance shopping trips to save gas. As a result, they are spending more at drug and convenience stores with big, easy-access candy sections. Then there's the "feel good" factor.

A dollar candy bar treat in the face of filling up the gas tank for nearly $100 can be a powerful psychological motivator," said James Russo, vice president of marketing for Nielsen's food sector. Candy's reputation for getting people through tough times is long-standing.

During the Great Depression, a nickel chocolate bar was sustenance. Some had names such as "Chicken Dinner."

Candy bars, during the Depression, were really America's fast food," said Steve Almond, author of "Candyfreak," a book that examines the economic history and allure of chocolate. "They were expressly **marketed** in a way that would suggest to people that **this was a cheap deal."** Such strategies helped some candy makers and sellers weather a weak economy.

One of them was the McKeesport Candy Co., a wholesaler in Pennsylvania that was established in 1927. Now the company does business on the Internet as Candyfavorites.com.

But even if consumers are willing to spend, this isn't an easy time for the candy industry, said Jon H. Prince, president of both companies.

Are we going to say that business is easier now that gas is $4 a gallon? Probably not," he said, citing such factors as the cost of transporting candy.

It's also a time when you're likely to see the biggest candy makers consolidating, much like the airline industry, said Pat Conroy, a consumer products expert at accounting and consulting firm Deloitte & Touche. The rising price of ingredients is part of the issue.

This year, the Hershey Co., one of the nation's biggest candy makers, raised its prices and announced job cuts and a plan to close several U.S. manufacturing plants, causing merger speculation.

And this spring, Mars Inc., the Virginia-based maker of M&Ms and Snickers, announced the purchase of Chicago's Wm. Wrigley Jr. Co., which is known for its Juicy Fruit and Doublemint gum, as well as Life Savers.

Unless you have a very powerful niche, the worst place you want to be is in the middle (in size)," Conroy said. "That's the danger zone." Still, he and others say the largest companies with dominant brands should do well, as will smaller specialty shops, which make the type of high end chocolate stay-at-home mom Nancy Bason seeks out.

A recent craving prompted her spontaneous visit to Sarah's Pastries & Candies, a storefront and kitchen in Chicago's Lincoln Park neighborhood that specializes in French-style chocolates.
"I don't buy chocolate every single day," said Bason, who lives nearby. "So if I'm treating myself once a week, it doesn't seem like I really need to cut back because it's not an everyday purchase."

She says she's much more likely to forgo the expensive latte, and is also holding back on buying clothing and big-ticket items such as appliances.

Back in Wisconsin, Towne has found his own way to deal with his sweet tooth, while trying to keep his candy budget in check. He's asking friends to sift through the discount bins at a local drugstore chain for boxes of Chewy Lemonhead & Friends, a new favorite that's a variation on a candy classic.

"Pathetic? Perhaps," Towne said of his cost-cutting tactics. "But oh so delicious."
business of candy is 'recession-proof'
* * * * * * * * * * * * * * * * * * *

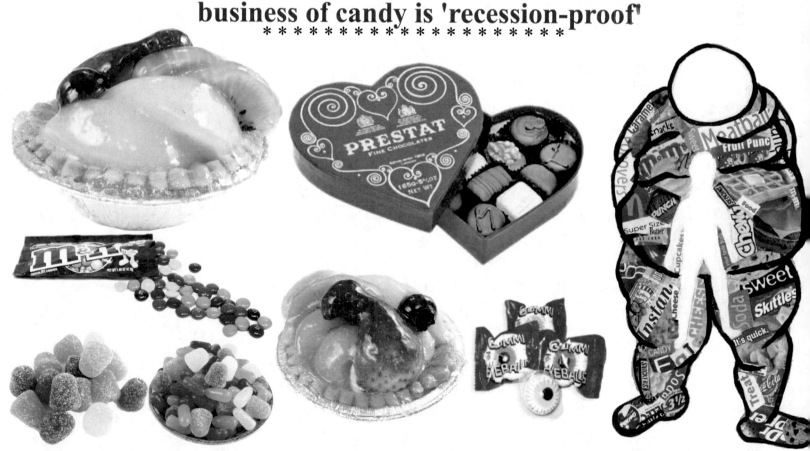

Wheaty Indiscretions:

What Happens to Wheat From Seed to Storage

Jen Allbritton, Certified Nutritionist

Wheat — America's grain of choice. Its hardy, glutenous consistency makes it practical for a variety of foodstuffs—cakes, breads, pastas, cookies, bagels, pretzels, and cereals that have been puffed, shredded, and shaped. This ancient grain can actually be very nutritious when it is grown and prepared in the appropriate manner. Unfortunately, the indiscretions inflicted by our modern farming techniques and milling practices have dramatically reduced the quality of the commercial wheat berry and the flour it makes. You might think, "Wheat is wheat, what can they do that makes commercial varieties so bad?" Listen up, because you are in for a surprise!

It was the cultivation of grains — members of the grass family — that made civilization possible. Since wheat is one of the oldest known grains, its cultivation is as old as civilization itself. Some accounts suggest that mankind has used this wholesome food since 10,000 to 15,000 years BC.

Upon opening Egyptian tombs archeologists discovered large earthenware jars full of wheat to "sustain" the Pharaohs in the afterlife. Hippocrates, the father of medicine, was said to recommend stone-ground flour for its beneficial effects on the digestive tract. Once humans figured out how to grind wheat, they discovered that when water is added it can be naturally fermented and turned into beer and expandable dough.

Botanists have identified almost 30,000 varieties of wheat, which are assigned to one of several classifications according to their planting schedule and nutrient composition, such as hard red winter, hard red spring, soft red winter, durum, hard white, and soft white. Spring wheat is planted in the spring, and winter wheat is planted in the fall and shoots up the next spring to mature that summer. Soft, hard, and durum (even harder) wheats are classified according to the strength of their kernel. This strength is a function of the protein-to-starch ratio in the endosperm (the starchy middle layer of the seed). Hard wheats contain less starch, leaving a stronger protein matrix.

With the advent of modern farming, the number of varieties of wheat in common use has been drastically reduced. Today, just a few varieties account for 90 percent of the wheat grown in the world. When grown in well-nourished, fertile soil, whole wheat is rich in vitamin E and B complex, many minerals, including calcium and iron, as well as omega-3 fatty acids. Proper growing and milling methods are necessary to preserve these nutrients and prevent rancidity.

Unfortunately, due to the indiscretions inflicted by contemporary farming and processing of modern wheat, many people have become intolerant or even allergic to this nourishing grain. These indiscretions include depletion of the soil through the use of chemical fertilizers, pesticides and other chemicals, high-heat milling, refining and improper preparation, such as extrusion.

Rather than focus on soil fertility and careful selection of seed to produce varieties tailored to a particular micro-climate, modern farming practices use high-tech methods to deal with pests and disease, leading to overdependence on chemicals and other substances.

It starts with the seed
Even before they are planted in the ground, wheat seeds receive an application of fungicides and insecticides. Fungicides are used to control diseases of seeds and seedlings; insecticides are used to control insect pests, killing them as they feed on the seed or emerging seedling. Seed companies often use mixtures of different seed-treatment fungicides or insecticides to control a broader spectrum of seed pests.

Pesticides and fertilizers
Some of the main chemicals (insecticides, herbicides and fungicides) used on commercial wheat crops are disulfoton (Di-syston), methyl parathion, chlorpyrifos, dimethoate, diamba and glyphosate. Although all these chemicals are approved for use and considered safe, consumers are wise to reduce their exposure as much as possible. Besides contributing to the overall toxic load in our bodies, these chemicals increase our susceptibility to neurotoxic diseases as well as to conditions like cancer. Many of these pesticides function as xenoestrogens, foreign estrogen that can reap havoc with our hormone balance and may be a contributing factor to a number of health conditions. For example, researchers speculate these estrogen-mimicking chemicals are one of the contributing factors to boys and girls entering puberty at earlier and earlier ages. They have also been linked to abnormalities and hormone-related cancers including fibrocystic breast disease, breast cancer and endometriosis.

Hormones on wheat?

Sounds strange, but farmers apply hormone-like substances or "plant growth regulators" that affect wheat characteristics, such as time of germination and strength of stalk. These hormones are either "natural," that is, extracted from other plants, or synthetic. Cycocel is a synthetic hormone that is commonly applied to wheat. Moreover, research is being conducted on how to manipulate the naturally occurring hormones in wheat and other grains to achieve "desirable" changes, such as regulated germination and an increased ability to survive in cold weather. No studies exist that isolate the health risks of eating hormone-manipulated wheat or varieties that have been exposed to hormone application. However, there is substantial evidence about the dangers of increasing our intake of hormone-like substances.

Chemicals used in storage

Chemical offenses don't stop after the growing process. The long storage of grains makes them vulnerable to a number of critters. Before commercial grain is even stored, the collection bins are sprayed with insecticide, inside and out. More chemicals are added while the bin is filled. These so-called "protectants" are then added to the upper surface of the grain as well as four inches deep into the grain to protect against damage from moths and other insects entering from the top of the bin. The list of various chemicals used includes chlorpyrifos-methyl, diatomaceous earth, bacillus thuringiensis, cy-fluthrin, malathion and pyrethrins. Then there is the threshold test. If there is one live insect per quart of sample, fumigation is initiated. The goal of fumigation is to "maintain a toxic concentration of gas long enough to kill the target pest population." The toxic chemicals penetrate the entire storage facility as well as the grains being treated. Two of the fumigants used include methyl bromide and phosphine-producing materials, such as magnesium phosphide or aluminum phosphide.

Grain drying

Heat damage is a serious problem that results from the artificial drying of damp grain at high temperatures. Overheating causes denaturing of the protein26 and can also partially cook the protein, ruining the flour's baking properties and nutritional value. According to Ed Lysenko, who tests grain by baking it into bread for the Canadian Grain Commission's grain research laboratory, wheat can be dried without damage by using re-circulating batch dryers, which keep the wheat moving during drying. He suggests an optimal drying temperature of 60 degrees Celsius (140 degrees Fahrenheit). Unfortunately, grain processors do not always take these precautions.

6

Modern processing

The damage inflicted on wheat does not end with cultivation and storage, but continues into milling and processing. A grain kernel is comprised of three layers: the bran, the germ and the endosperm. The bran is the outside layer where most of the fiber exists. The germ is the inside layer where many nutrients and essential fatty acids are found. The endosperm is the starchy middle layer. The high nutrient density associated with grains exists only when these three are intact. The term whole grain refers to the grain before it has been milled into flour. It was not until the late nineteenth century that white bread, biscuits, and cakes made from white flour and sugars became mainstays in the diets of industrialized nations, and these products were only made possible with the invention of high-speed milling machines. Dr. Price observed the unmistakable consequences of these dietary changes during his travels and documented their corresponding health effects. These changes not only resulted in tooth decay, but problems with fertility, mental health and disease progression.

Flour was originally produced by grinding grains between large stones. The final product, 100 percent stone-ground whole-wheat flour, contained everything that was in the grain, including the germ, fiber, starch and a wide variety of vitamins and minerals. Without refrigeration or chemical preservatives, fresh stone-ground flour spoils quickly. After wheat has been ground, natural wheat-germ oil becomes rancid at about the same rate that milk becomes sour, so refrigeration of whole grain breads and flours is necessary. Technology's answer to these issues has been to apply faster, hotter and more aggressive processing.

Since grinding stones are not fast enough for mass-production, the industry uses high-speed, steel roller mills that eject the germ and the bran. Much of this "waste product"—the most nutritious part of the grain—is sold as "byproducts" for animals. The resulting white flour contains only a fraction of the nutrients of the original grain. Even whole wheat flour is compromised during the modern milling process. High-speed mills reach 400 degrees Fahrenheit, and this heat destroys vital nutrients and creates rancidity in the bran and the germ. Vitamin E in the germ is destroyed — a real tragedy because whole wheat used to be our most readily available source of vitamin E.

Literally dozens of dough conditioners and preservatives go into modern bread, as well as toxic ingredients like partially hydrogenated vegetable oils and soy flour. Soy flour — loaded with anti-nutrients — is added to virtually all brand-name breads today to improve rise and prevent sticking. The extrusion process, used to make cold breakfast cereals and puffed grains, adds insult to injury with high temperatures and high pressures that create additional toxic components and further destroy nutrients — even the synthetic vitamins that are added to replace the ones destroyed by refinement and milling.

People have become accustomed to the mass-produced, gooey, devitalized, and nutritionally deficient breads and baked goods and have little recollection of how real bread should taste. Chemical preservatives allow bread to be shipped long distances and to remain on the shelf for many days without spoiling and without refrigeration.

Healthy whole wheat products

Ideally, one should buy whole wheat berries and grind them fresh to make homemade breads and other baked goods. Buy whole wheat berries that are grown organically or biodynamically — biodynamic farming involves higher standards than organic. Since these forms of farming do not allow synthetic, carcinogenic chemicals and fertilizers, purchasing organic or biodynamic wheat assures that you are getting the cleanest, most nutritious food possible. It also automatically eliminates the possibility of irradiation and genetically engineered seed. The second best option is to buy organic 100 percent stone-ground whole-wheat flour at a natural food store. Slow-speed, steel hammer-mills are often used instead of stones, and flours made in this way can list "stone-ground" on the label. This method is equivalent to the stone-ground process and produces a product that is equally nutritious. Any process that renders the entire grain into usable flour without exposing it to high heat is acceptable.

If you do not make your own bread, there are ready-made alternatives available. Look for organic sourdough or sprouted breads freshly baked or in the freezer compartment of your market or health food store. If bread is made entirely with 100 percent stone-ground whole grains, it will state so on the label. When bread is stone ground and then baked, the internal temperature does not usually exceed 170 degrees, so most of the nutrients are preserved. As they contain no preservatives, both whole wheat flour and its products should be kept in the refrigerator or freezer. Stone-ground flour will keep for several months frozen.

Sprouting, soaking and genuine sourdough leavening "pre-digests" grains, allowing the nutrient to be more easily assimilated and metabolized. This is an age-old approach practiced in most traditional cultures. Sprouting begins germination, which increases the enzymatic activity in foods and inactivates substances called enzyme inhibitors. These enzyme inhibitors prevent the activation of the enzymes present in the food and, therefore, may hinder optimal digestion and absorption. Soaking neutralizes phytic acid, a component of plant fiber found in the bran and hulls of grains, legumes, nuts, and seeds that reduces mineral absorption. All of these benefits may explain why sprouted foods are less likely to produce allergic reactions in those who are sensitive.

 Sprouting also causes a beneficial modification of various nutritional elements. According to research undertaken at the University of Minnesota, sprouting increases the total nutrient density of a food. For example, sprouted whole wheat was found to have 28 percent more thiamine (B1), 315 percent more riboflavin (B2), 66 percent more niacin (B3), 65 percent more pantothenic acid (B5), 111 percent more biotin, 278 percent more folic acid, and 300 percent more vitamin C than non-sprouted whole wheat. This phenomenon is not restricted to wheat. All grains undergo this type of quantitative and qualitative transformation. These studies also confirmed a significant increase in enzymes, which means the nutrients are easier to digest and absorb.

You have several options for preparing your wheat. You can use a sour leavening method by mixing whey, buttermilk or yogurt with freshly ground wheat or quality pre-ground wheat from the store. Or, soak your berries whole for 8 to 22 hours, then drain and rinse. There are some recipes that use the whole berries while they are wet, such as cracker dough ground right in the food processor. Another option is to dry sprouted wheat berries in a low-temperature oven or dehydrator, and then grind them in your grain mill and then use the flour in a variety or recipes. Although our modern wheat suffers from a great number of indiscretions, there are steps we can take to find the quality choices that will nourish us today and for the long haul. Go out and make a difference for you and yours and turn your wheaty indiscretions into wheaty indulgences.

* * * * * * * * * * * * * * * * * * * *

No-Nos!

reads, cake, pie, cookies, candy, pancakes, waffles, flour tortillas, puddings tore-bought), cereals and any processed foods, all contribute to being verweight.

oods containing white flour and white sugar. Sodas, wines, beer, hard quor, breaded foods, syrups, canned fruit, coffee, any "empty" calories, tificial sweeteners, and white rice. Watch out too, for high-fructose corn yrup, and related sugars, ice cream, pizza, pasta, and jello. Preservatives: trites, sulfites also need to be crossed off your nutritional list.

Okay Foods

ll fruits and vegetables, avocados, olives, eggs, meat, fish, poultry, nuts, orn tortillas, soups, 100% whole grain wheat, brown rice, barley, uckwheat, etc. (This does not mean bread.)

ummy foods like 100% natural peanut butter (pour off the oil) and pplesauce, are fine, along with beans, olive oil, butter, cheese, water, and pioca.

s to: corn, brown rice and potatoes, use sparingly. Be sure to remove all fat om the meat before cooking.

ou can add more to this list as you learn more about nutrition and the foods n which your body truly thrives.

Bad Food Choices

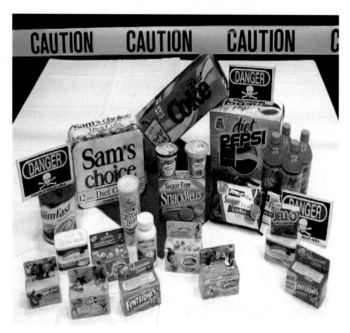

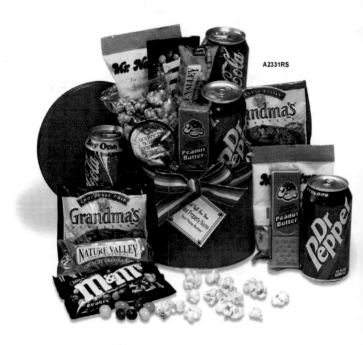

Good Food Choices

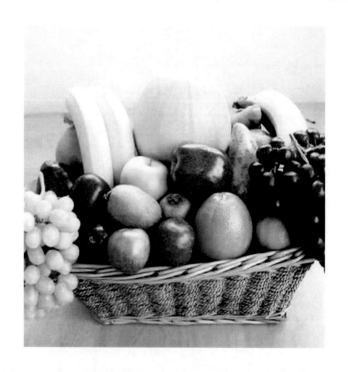

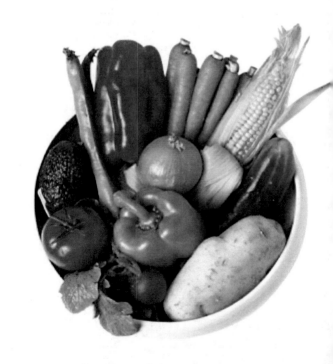

General Eating Guidelines

☞ Don't eat fatty foods.

☞ Don't eat any foods you don't like.

☞ Don't eat any foods that disagree with you.

☞ Don't eat foods to which you are allergic.

☞ Don't eat food just because it's been given to you, like at a party or at work, or school.

☞ Don't stuff yourself at the restaurant! Eat less and save money on your next meal — take half of your meal home in a doggie bag.

☞ Don't eat food combinations that disturb your body.

☞ Don't eat questionable food — if you have any doubt as to its source, age content, who handled it, etc.

☞ Don't drink liquids with your meals. Fluids taken with your meal can dilute the hormones in your digestive fluids.

☞ Don't eat to comfort yourself when you are upset.

☞ Don't eat just because you're lonely.

☞ Don't eat because of disappointments — exercise instead.

☞ Don't overeat when you're with other people. Be aware — the tendency is to eat more.

☞ Don't overeat any time. Make smaller portions for yourself and eat slowly.

DO eat only good food and when you are truly hungry!

What is Fiber?

Fiber Free for All ?
Not all fibers are equal

What Is Fiber?

Nobody knows! That's right, nobody knows exactly what fiber is. Scientist can' agree on a definition of fiber or even on how to measure the amount of it in food. I that isn't bad enough, we also aren't sure what it does. With all the confusion , how come nutritionists are so sure we should eat it—and why should you believe them'. Fruits and vegetables seem to fill the bill for fiber requirements.

The basic idea of fiber is that there are substances in some foods which cannot be digested and therefore pass through the intestine out into the feces. Obviously, if a substance passes right through like that, it won't supply the nutrients that your body needs.

Types of Fiber and Their Benefits

There are two types of fiber: insoluble and soluble. They both aid digestion and help you maintain a healthy weight. Foods rich in fiber are low in calories and fat, and fil' you up more. They may also reduce your risks for certain health problems.

Insoluble Fiber:

This is found in whole grains, cereals, certain fruits and vegetables (such as apple skin, corn, and carrots). Insoluble fiber: May prevent constipation—May reduce the risk of certain types of cancer.

Soluble Fiber:

This type of fiber is in oats, beans and certain fruits and vegetables (such as strawberries and peas). Soluble fiber: Can reduce cholesterol, which may help lower the risk of heart disease—Helps control blood sugar levels.

LOOK FOR HIGH FIBER FOODS

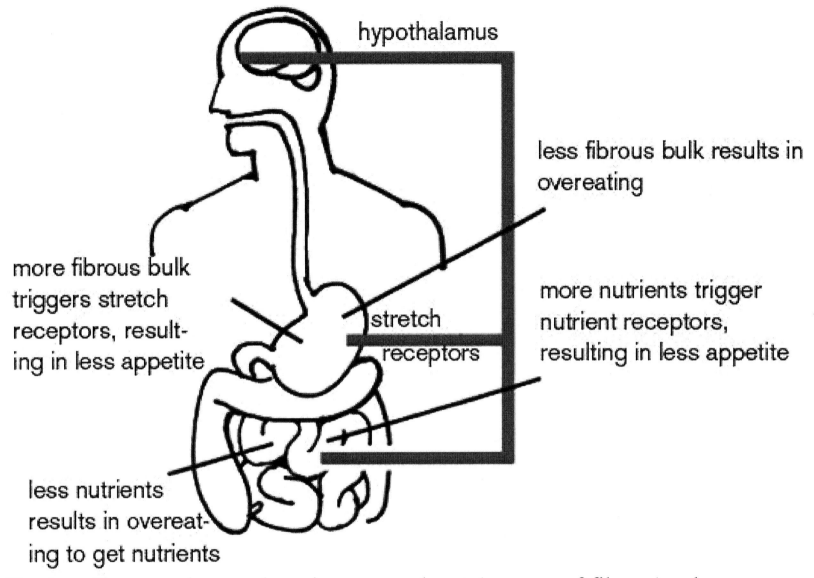

Fruits– Two servings a day give you at least 4 grams of fiber. Apples, oranges, strawberries, pears, and bananas are good sources.

Vegetables—Three servings a day give you at least 6 grams of fiber. Add asparagus, carrots, broccoli, peas, and corn to your meals.

Legumes—One serving a day in place of meat gives you at least 4 grams of fiber. Try navy beans, lentils, and chickpeas.

Seeds—A small handful of seeds gives you about 3 grams of fiber. Try sunflower seeds.

Companies Sued for Carcinogens in Food

August 2, 2008

LOS ANGELES – Four food manufacturers have agreed to reduce levels of a cancer-causing chemical in their **potato chips and french** fries in a settlement with the state of California.

The state attorney general's office announced the deals yesterday with **Heinz, Frito-Lay, Kettle Foods and Lance Inc.**

The lawsuits were filed under a state law that requires companies to post warnings about carcinogens in their products.

The attorney general's office sued the manufacturers and several fast food companies in 2005 **because their products contained high levels of acrylamide.** The office said the companies agreed to lower the levels and pay a combined $3 million in fines.

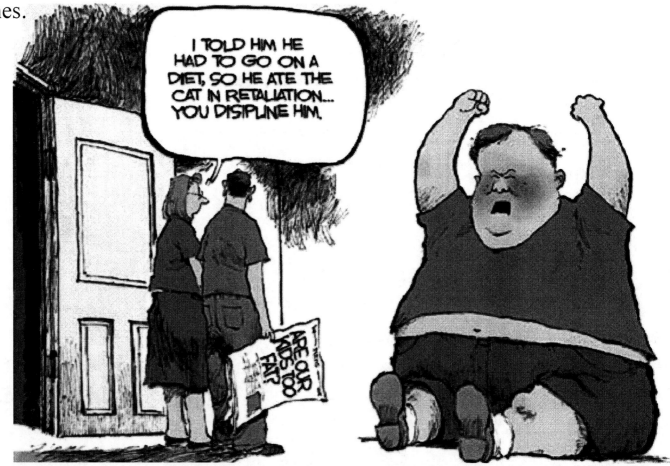

For the Children

child's total diet, and his or her activity level, both play an important role in determining child's weight. Our kids are getting set up now for problems with obesity, heart disease, abetes or cancer, later on in life. Our number one objective should be to find ways to get kids tive and fit. Our schools need to be creative in making physical education fun and informative. 'e need to teach life skills, not just how to run laps. The societies of the world are beginning to alize that exercise and physical education are important to the complete individual as in dy, mind, and soul.

Excerpted from a paper by Peter J. Manosh, MBA;
leading authority in food science, human nutrition, exercise and sport science.

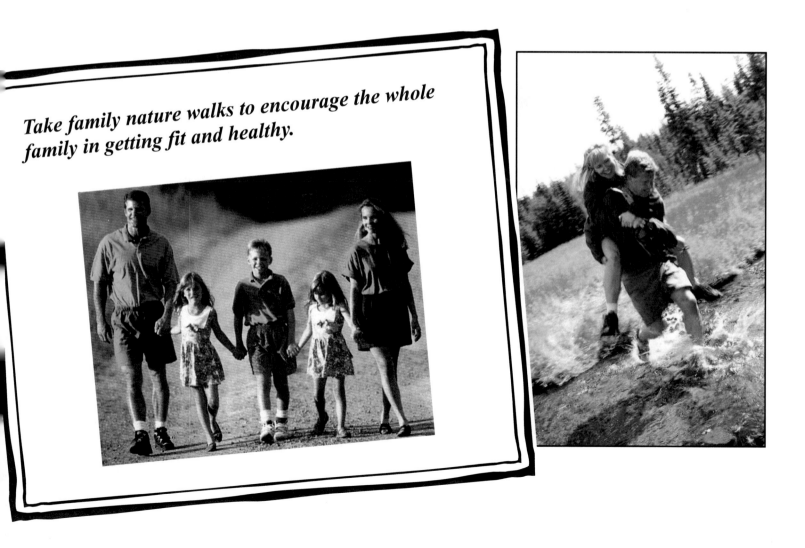

Take family nature walks to encourage the whole family in getting fit and healthy.

Center for Science in the Public Interest (CSPI, www.cspinet.org)

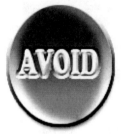 Unsafe in amounts consumed or is very poorly tested and not worth any risk.

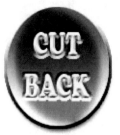 Not toxic, but large amou... may be unsafe or promote bad nutrition.

-ACESULFAME POTASSIUM
-ARTIFICIAL COLORINGS (BLUE 1, BLUE 2, GREEN 3, RED 3, YELLOW 6)
-ASPARTAME (NutraSweet)
-BUTYLATED HYDROXYANISOLE (BHA)
-CYCLAMATE
(not legal in U.S.)
-HYDROGENATED VEGETABLE OIL
-OLESTRA (Olean)
-PARTIALLY HYDROGENATED VEGETABLE OIL
-POTASSIUM BROMATE
-PROPYL GALLATE
-SACCHARIN
-SODIUM NITRITE
-STEVIA

-CAFFEINE
-CORN SYRUP
-DEXTROSE (CORN SUGAR, GLUCOSE)
-HIGH-FRUCTOSE CORN SYRUP
-HYDROGENATED STARCH HYDROLYSATE
-INVERT SUGAR
-LACTITOL
-MALTITOL
-POLYDEXTROSE
-SALATRIM
-SALT
-SORBITOL
-SUGAR
-TAGATOSE

Center for Science in the Public Interest (CSPI, www.cspinet.org)

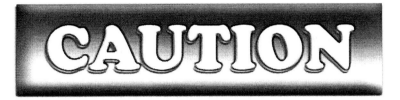

May pose a risk and needs to be better tested.

-ARTIFICIAL COLORINGS (CITRUS RED, RED 40)
-BROMINATED VEGETABLE OIL (BVO)
-BUTYLATED HYDROXYTOLUENE (BHT)
-DIACETYL
-HEPTYL PARABEN
-QUININE

-ARTIFICIAL COLORINGS (YELLOW 5)
-ARTIFICIAL AND NATURAL FLAVORING
-BETA-CAROTENE
-CAFFEINE
-CARMINE
-COCHINEAL
-CASEIN
-GUM TRAGACANTH
-HVP (HYDROLYZED VEGETABLE PROTEIN)
-LACTOSE
-MSG (MONOSODIUM GLUTAMATE)
-MYCOPROTEIN
-QUININE
-SODIUM BENZOATE
-SODIUM BISULFITE
-SULFITES
-SULFUR DIOXIDE

Center for Science in the Public Interest (CSPI, www.cspinet.org)

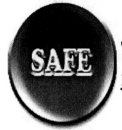 **The additive *appears* to be safe. (Author: But not necessarily so, and more thorough investigation is needed.)**

-ALGINATE
-ALPHA TOCOPHEROL (Vitamin E)
-ASCORBIC ACID
(Vitamin C)
-BETA-CAROTENE
-CALCIUM PROPIONATE
-CALCIUM STEAROYL LACTYLATE
-CARRAGEENAN
-CASEIN
-CITRIC ACID
-DIACYLGLYCEROL
-EDTA
-ERYTHORBIC ACID
-FERROUS GLUCONATE
-FUMARIC ACID
-GELATIN
-GLYCERIN (Glycerol)
-GUMS: Arabic, Furcelleran, Ghatti,
Guar, Karaya,
Locust Bean, Xanthan
-LACTIC ACID
-LECITHIN
-MONO- and DIGLYCERIDES

-NEOTAME
-OLIGOFRUCTOSE
-TRIACETIN (GLYCEROL
TRIACETATE)
-VANILLIN, ETHYL VANILLIN
-VEGETABLE OIL STEROL ESTERS-
PHOSPHATE SALTS
-PHOSPHORIC ACID
-PLANT STEROLS AND STANOLS
-POLYSORBATE 60, 65, 80
-POTASSIUM SORBATE
-PROPYLENE GLYCOL ALGINATE
-SODIUM ASCORBATE
-SODIUM CARBOXY-
METHYLCELLULOSE (CMC)
-SODIUM CASEINATE
-SODIUM CITRATE
-SODIUM PROPIONATE
-SODIUM STEAROYL LACTYLATE
-SORBIC ACID
-SORBITAN MONOSTEARATE
-STARCH, MODIFIED STARCH
-SUCRALOSE
-THIAMIN MONONITRATE

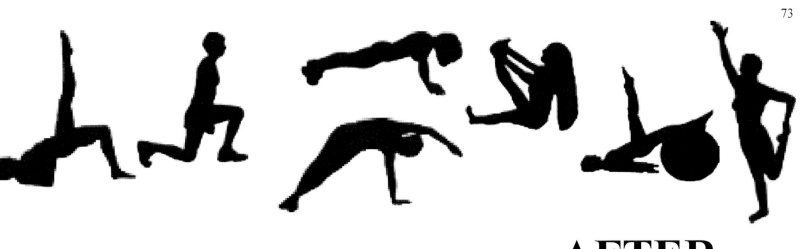

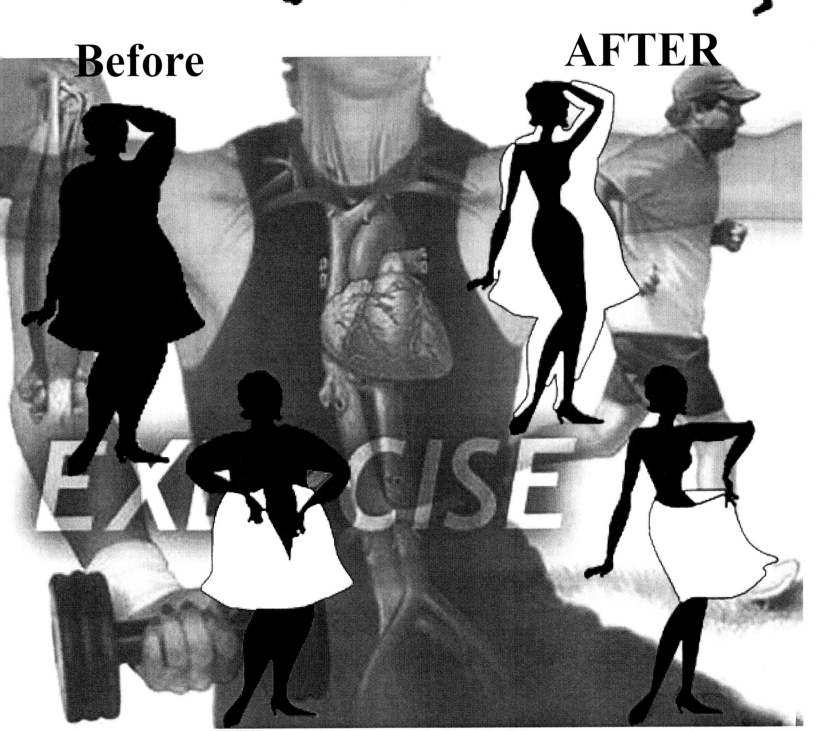

Before

AFTER

"ONE exercise fits all? Not by any stretch"

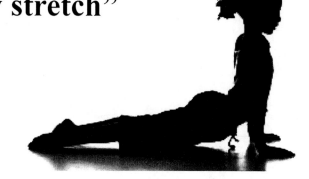

By Diane Suchetka
Newhouse News Service/*San Diego Union-Tribune*
June 17, 2008

Boy, can we pave the road to hell.

We work so hard at getting fit, we hurt ourselves. And we find a thousand ways to do it.

We skip warm-ups, forget to stretch, think posture doesn't matter. And we ignore that pain in ou
knee for weeks. (It'll go away, won't it?)

Then reality hits us — often in the physical therapist's office.

Here's the problem: Most exercise advice is designed for the perfectly healthy, perfectly normal
perfectly fit human being. And we all know nobody's perfect.

"What it all boils down to is everybody's body is very specific in how it moves and how it's pu
together," says Ed Baldwin, a physical therapist in Ohio. "So exercise programs need to be
structured around the individual.

"We all need to seek professional advice specifically designed for us."

That's especially true if we've been injured or have chronic pain in a joint or some other health
concern.

Even the old standbys, the simple exercises that are supposed to be good for everybody,
sometimes can do more harm than good.

"I don't want to discourage anyone from walking," Baldwin says. "But it can irritate a hip
problem. It can make a back problem worse. It can irritate knees.
"And swimming can irritate the shoulders and lower back."

So what do you do? A few simple steps will get you on the right track.

The first one: See your doctor before you start a new exercise program. Once you get the OK, keep three basics in mind:

Warm up: It's crucial. Length and intensity should vary, depending on your sport and fitness level. Typically 10 to 15 minutes of brisk walking, bicycling or using an elliptical machine will do just fine.

"In general, a warm-up helps to elevate your heart rate, loosen up your muscles and warm up your body in preparation for strenuous activity," says Sara Pesut, also a physical therapist.

Stand up straight: Posture is critical when it comes to exercise. But all you have to do is follow the simple formula of keeping your body aligned – your ears squarely over your shoulders, shoulders over your hips, hips over your knees, knees over your feet.

When your body's balanced, your muscles don't waste energy. That means all of it goes to performance.

"And if you don't do an exercise in the correct posture, the mechanics are going to be off, increasing your chances of injury," Pesut says.

Cool down: This is another important aspect of exercise. Ten minutes or so of slow jogging or walking decelerates your heart rate and prevents lactic acid buildup and cramping.

If you really want to stay off the injured list, consider the most consistent piece of advice from physical therapists: Talk to someone who can coach you one-on-one.

"That ensures that you'll have a comprehensive program and that you won't be missing parts of your routine," says Gary Calabrese, director of Sports Health and Orthopaedic Rehabilitation at the Cleveland Clinic. "And a comprehensive program, with all the necessary components, maximizes your athletic performance – you'll be able to get strong faster."
You'll also reduce your chances of injury.

And that will keep you from getting frustrated and ditching your routine altogether.

Of course, Pesut says, you need to do your homework and check credentials. "Maybe even ask for a referral," she says.

Start, once again, with your doctor. Or check with longtime athletes in your field who know who's good and who's not.

You also can schedule an appointment to see a licensed physical therapist. They are the experts who will fix you if you get hurt, so why not consult them before it happens?

Often, only one or two sessions are necessary. And doctors often are willing to write prescriptions for the service so your insurance covers it. Check your plan; you may not even need a referral.

"It's not hard for any experienced physical therapist to help you in that regard," Baldwin says. "In one session, I can determine where an individual's problems lie in regards to flexibility and posture and get them going on the right fitness program."

In the end, it'll keep you off the bench.

And, as Calabrese says: "The best injury is the one that's prevented."

**DON'T TRY TO BE AN ARNOLD!
LIGHT WEIGHT TRAINING WITH A VARIETY OF
CARDIOVASCULAR EXERCISES WILL HELP YOU
ACHIEVE A PHYSICAL FITNESS**

Why Did Tim Die ?

They say it was a heart attack but looking at his obituary it's found that he was overweight and had diabetes. What a shame that a highly respected, intelligent journalist would be taken at such an early age. It was a great loss.

What Tim died of was really diet mismanagement, and ignorance of how to live a lifestyle that vessels in good health!

hope that a new movement in his honor for better education for better health.

There are over 300,000 Tims and Marys in our country that die annually of heart diseases.

Don't you think it is diet mismanagement?

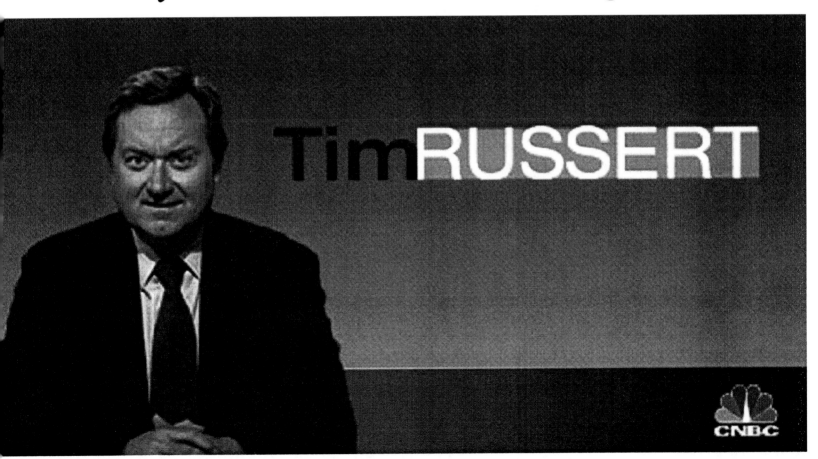

Evolution

The Obituaries are Full of "Heart"-Aches
Poor diets can affect length of life

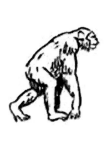
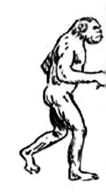

No one is immune to dying. It will happen to all of us. Some sooner than later and we can prolong the event, with a lifestyle change of healthy eating and proper exercise. But even our leaders and experts succumb to poor diet habits and inactivity. Health checkups are also vitally important, to diagnose problems early enough to treat.

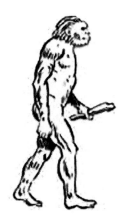
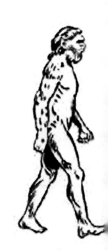

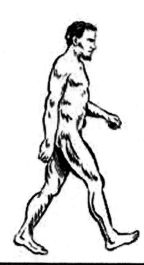
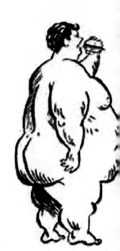

144 Reasons Why Sugar Is Ruining Your Health
Nancy Appleton, Ph.D.

. Sugar can suppress the immune system.

2. Sugar upsets the mineral relationships in the body.

. Sugar can cause hyperactivity, anxiety, difficulty concentrating, and crankiness in children.

4. Sugar can produce a significant rise in triglycerides.

5. Sugar contributes to the reduction in defense against bacterial infection (infectious diseases).

6. Sugar causes a loss of tissue elasticity and function, the more sugar you eat the more elasticity and function you loose.

7. Sugar reduces high-density lipoproteins.

8. Sugar leads to chromium deficiency.

9. Sugar leads to cancer of the ovaries.

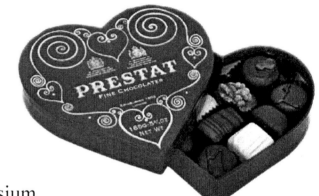

10. Sugar can increase fasting levels of glucose.

11. Sugar causes copper deficiency.

12. Sugar interferes with absorption of calcium and magnesium.

13. Sugar may make eyes more vulnerable to age-related macular degeneration.

14. Sugar raises the level of a neurotransmitters: dopamine, serotonin, and norepinephrine.

15. Sugar can cause hypoglycemia.

16. Sugar can produce an acidic digestive tract.

17. Sugar can cause a rapid rise of adrenaline levels in children.

18. Sugar malabsorption is frequent in patients with functional bowel disease.

19. Sugar can cause premature aging.

20. Sugar can lead to alcoholism.

21. Sugar can cause tooth decay.

22. Sugar contributes to obesity

23. High intake of sugar increases the risk of Crohn's disease, and ulcerative colitis.

24. Sugar can cause changes frequently found in person with gastric or duodenal ulcers.

25. Sugar can cause arthritis.

26. Sugar can cause asthma.

27. Sugar greatly assists the uncontrolled growth of Candida Albicans (yeast infections).

28. Sugar can cause gallstones.

29. Sugar can cause heart disease.

30. Sugar can cause appendicitis.

31. Sugar can cause hemorrhoids.

32. Sugar can cause varicose veins.

33. Sugar can elevate glucose and insulin responses in oral contraceptive users.

34. Sugar can lead to periodontal disease.

35. Sugar can contribute to osteoporosis.

36. Sugar contributes to saliva acidity.

37. Sugar can cause a decrease in insulin sensitivity.

38. Sugar can lower the amount of Vitamin E (alpha-Tocopherol) in the blood.

39. Sugar can decrease growth hormone.

40. Sugar can increase cholesterol.

41. Sugar can increase the systolic blood pressure.

42. High sugar intake increases advanced glycation end products (AGEs, Sugar bound non-enzymatically to protein)

43. Sugar can interfere with the absorption of protein.

44. Sugar causes food allergies.

45. Sugar can contribute to diabetes.

46. Sugar can cause toxemia during pregnancy.

47. Sugar can contribute to eczema in children.

48. Sugar can cause cardiovascular disease.

49. Sugar can impair the structure of DNA

50. Sugar can change the structure of protein.

51. Sugar can make our skin age by changing the structure of collagen.
52. Sugar can cause cataracts.
53. Sugar can cause emphysema.
54. Sugar can cause atherosclerosis.
55. Sugar can promote an elevation of low-density lipoproteins (LDL).
56. High sugar intake can impair the physiological homeostasis of many systems in the body.
57. Sugar lowers the enzymes ability to function.
58. Sugar intake is higher in people with Parkinson's disease.
59. Sugar can increase the size of the liver by making the liver cells divide.
60. Sugar can increase the amount of liver fat.
61. Sugar can increase kidney size and produce pathological changes in the kidney.
62. Sugar can damage the pancreas.
63. Sugar can increase the body's fluid retention.
64. Sugar is enemy #1 of the bowel movement.
65. Sugar can cause myopia (nearsightedness).
66. Sugar can compromise the lining of the capillaries.
67. Sugar can make the tendons more brittle.
68. Sugar can cause headaches, including migraine.
69. Sugar plays a role in pancreatic cancer in women.
70. Sugar can adversely affect school children's grades and cause learning disorders.
71. Sugar can cause depression.
72. Sugar increases the risk of gastric cancer.
73. Sugar and cause dyspepsia (indigestion).
74. Sugar can increase your risk of getting gout.
75. Sugar can increase the levels of glucose in an oral glucose tolerance test over the ingestion of complex carbohydrates.

76. Sugar can increase the insulin responses in humans consuming high-sugar diets compared to low-sugar diets.

77. A diet high in refined sugar reduces learning capacity.

78. Sugar can cause less effective functioning of two blood proteins, albumin, and lipoproteins, which may reduce the body's ability to handle fat and cholesterol.

79. Sugar can contribute to Alzheimer's disease.

80. Sugar can cause platelet adhesiveness.

81. Sugar can cause hormonal imbalance; some hormones become under active and others become overactive.

82. Sugar can lead to the formation of kidney stones.

83. Diets high in sugar can cause free radicals and oxidative stress.

84. High sugar diet can lead to biliary tract cancer.

85. High sugar consumption of pregnant adolescents is associated with a twofold-increased risk for delivering a small-for-gestational-age (SGA) infant.

86. High sugar consumption can lead to substantial decrease in gestation duration among adolescents.

87. Sugar slows food's travel time through the gastrointestinal tract.

88. Sugar increases the concentration of bile acids in stools and bacterial enzymes in the colon. This can modify bile to produce cancer-causing compounds and colon cancer.

89. Sugar increases estradiol (the most potent form of naturally occurring estrogen) in men.

90. Sugar combines with and destroys phosphatase, an enzyme, which makes the process of digestion more difficult.

91. Sugar can be a risk factor of gallbladder cancer.

92. Sugar is an addictive substance.

93. Sugar can be intoxicating, similar to alcohol.

94. Sugar can exacerbate PMS.

95. Sugar given to premature babies can affect the amount of carbon dioxide they produce.

96. Decrease in sugar intake can increase emotional stability.

97. The rapid absorption of sugar promotes excessive food intake in obese subjects.

98. Sugar can worsen the symptoms of children with attention deficit hyperactivity disorder (ADHD).

99. Sugar adversely affects urinary electrolyte composition.

100. Sugar can slow down the ability of the adrenal glands to function.

101. IVs (intravenous feedings) of sugar water can cut off oxygen to the brain.

102. High sucrose intake could be an important risk factor in lung cancer.

103. Sugar increases the risk of polio.

104. High sugar intake can cause epileptic seizures.

105. Sugar causes high blood pressure in obese people.

106. In Intensive Care Units, limiting sugar saves lives.

107. Sugar may induce cell death.

108. Sugar can increase the amount of food that you eat.

109. In juvenile rehabilitation camps, when children were put on a low sugar diet, there was a 44% drop in antisocial behavior.

110. Sugar can lead to prostrate cancer.

111. Sugar dehydrates newborns.

112. Sugar can cause low birth weight babies.

113. Greater consumption of refined sugar is associated with a worse outcome of schizophrenia.

114. Sugar can raise homocysteine levels in the blood stream.

115. Sweet food items increase the risk of breast cancer.

116. Sugar is a risk factor in cancer of the small intestine.

117. Sugar may cause laryngeal cancer.

118. Sugar induces salt and water retention.

119. Sugar may contribute to mild memory loss.

120. The more sodas a 10 year old child consumes, the less milk.

121. Sugar can increase the total amount of food consumed.

122. Exposing a newborn to sugar results in a heightened preference for sucrose relative to water at 6 months and 2 years of age.

123. Sugar causes constipation.

124. Sugar causes varicose veins.

125. Sugar can cause brain decay in pre-diabetic and diabetic women.

126. Sugar can increase the risk of stomach cancer. 127. Sugar can cause metabolic syndrome.

128. Sugar ingestion by pregnant women increases neural tube defects in embryos.

129. Sugar can be a factor in asthma.

130. The higher the sugar consumption the more chances of getting irritable bowel syndrome.

131. Sugar can affect the brain's ability to deal with rewards and consequences.

132. Sugar can cause cancer of the rectum.

133. Sugar can cause endometrial cancer.

134. Sugar can cause renal (kidney) cell carcinoma.

135. Sugar can cause liver tumors.

136. Sugar can increase inflammatory markers in the blood stream of overweight people.

137. Sugar can lower Vitamin E levels in the blood stream.

138. Sugar can increase your appetite for all food.

139. Sugar plays a role in the etiology and the continuation of acne.

140. Too much sugar can kill your sex life.

141. Sugar saps school performance in children.

142. Sugar can cause fatigue, moodiness, nervousness and depression.

143. Sugar is common choice of obese individuals.

144. A linear decrease in the intake of many essential nutrients is associated with increasing total sugar intake.

85

The Eight Essential Biological Sugars

(from table sugar)

1 Glucose

Typically, only these two are found in our modern diets

2 Galactose

(from milk products)

3 Mannose

4 Xylose

5 Fucose

6 N-Acetyl-glucosamine

7 N-Acetyl-galactosamine

8 N-Acetyl-neuraminic acid

85

The Top 20 Worst Restaurant Foods in America!
(Countdown from 20 to the #1 worst!)

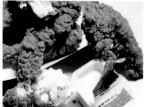

20: McDonald's (5 pieces) with creamy ranch sauce · 830 calories · 55 grams (g) fat (4.5g trans fat) · 48g carbohydrates

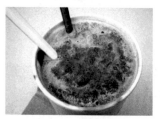

19: Worst drink **Jamba Juice Chocolate Moo'd Power Smoothie (30 fl oz)** · 900 calories 10g fat · 183g carbs (166g sugar)

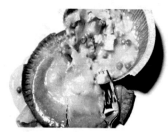

18: Worst supermarket meal **Pepperidge Farm Roasted Chicken Pot Pie (whole pie)** · 1,020 calories 64 g fat · 86g carbs

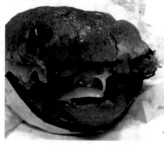

17: Worst "healthy" burger **Ruby Tuesday Bella Turkey Burger** · 1,145 calories 71g fat · 56g carbs

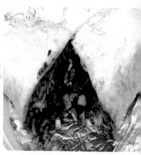

16: Worst Mexic entrée **Chipotle Mexican Grill Chicken Burrit** 1,179 calories 47 fat · 125g carbs 2,656 milligrams (mg) sodium

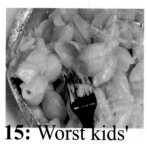

15: Worst kids' meal **Macaroni Grill Double Macaroni 'n' Cheese** · 1,210 calories 62g fat · 3,450 mg sodium

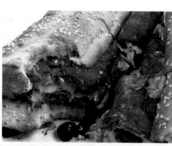

14: Worst sandwich **Quiznos Classic Italian (large)** · 1,490 calories 85g fat · 4,510 mg sodium 96g carbs

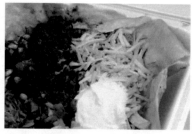

13: Worst salad **On the Border Grande Taco Salad with Taco Beef** · 1,450 calories 102g fat · 78g carbs 2,410mg sodium

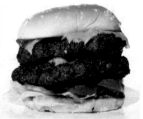

12: Worst burger **Carl's Jr. Double Six Dollar Burger** · 1,520 calories · 111g fat

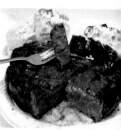

11: Worst steak **Lonestar 20 oz T-bone** · 1,540 calorie · 124g fat

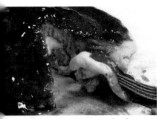

**: Worst breakfast
ob Evans
aramel Banana
ecan Cream
acked and
uffed Hotcakes**
1,540 calories ·
7g fat (9g trans
t)· 198g carbs
09g sugar)

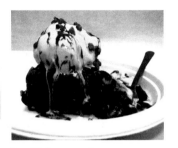

9: Worst dessert
**Chili's Chocolate
Chip Paradise Pie
with Vanilla Ice
Cream** · 1,600
calories · 78g fat·
215g carbs

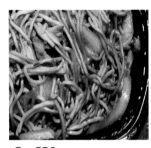

8: Worst
Chinese entrée
**P.F. Chang's
Pork Lo Mein**·
1,820 calories ·
127g fat· 95g
carbs

7: Worst chicken
entrée **Chili's
Honey Chipotle
Crispers with
Chipotle Sauce**
· 2,040 calories
· 99g fat · 240g
carbs

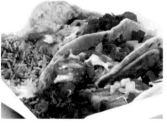

6: Worst fish
entrée **On the
Border Dos XX
Fish Tacos with
Rice and Beans**
· 2,100 calories
· 130g fat·
169g carbs
4,750mg sodium

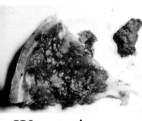

: Worst pizza
**Jno Chicago
Grill Chicago
Classic Deep
Dish Pizza** ·
,310 calories ·
62g fat· 123g
arbs· 4,470mg
odium

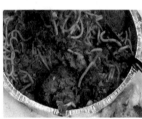

4: Worst pasta
**Macaroni
Grill Spaghetti
and Meatballs
with Meat
Sauce** · 2,430
calories · 128g
fat · 207g carbs
· 5,290mg
sodium

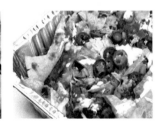

3: Worst
nachos **On the
Border
Stacked
Border
Nachos** ·
2,740 calories ·
166g fat 191g
carbs ·
5,280mg

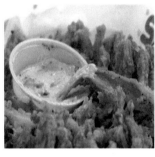

2: Worst starter
**Chili's Awesome
Blossom** · 2,710
calories · 203g
fat· 194g carbs ·
6,360mg sodium

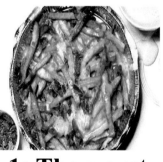

**1: The worst
food in
America**
**Outback
Steakhouse
Aussie Cheese
Fries with
Ranch Dressing**
· 2,900 calories
· 182g fat·
240g carbs

Nature's Design

So the real question is, why do we trust in drugs and doctors when the simple answers are found in nature?

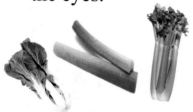

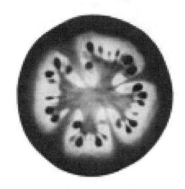

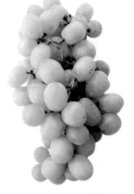

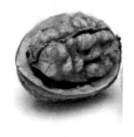

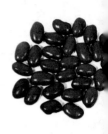

A **sliced carrot** looks like the **human eye** — the pupil, iris and radiating lines look just like the human eye …carrots greatly enhance blood flow to and function of the eyes.

A **tomato** has four chambers and is red. **The heart** tomatoes are indeed pure heart and blood food.

Grapes hang in a cluster that has the shape of **the heart**. grapes are also profound heart and blood vitalizing food.

A **walnut** looks like a **little brain**, We now know that walnuts help develop over 3 dozen neuron-transmitters for brain function.

Kidney Beans actually heal and help maintain kidney function and yes, they look exactly like the human kidneys.

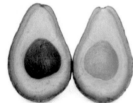

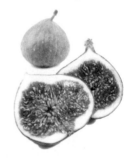

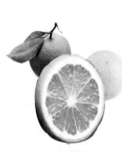

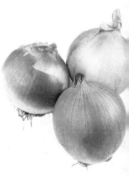

Celery, Bok Choy, Rhubarb and more, look just like **bones**. These foods specifically target bone strength. These foods replenish the skeletal needs of the body.

Eggplant, Avocadoes and **Pears** target the health and function of the **womb** and **cervix** of the female — they look just like these organs. … It takes exactly *9 months to grow an avocado* from blossom to ripened fruit.

Figs are full of seeds and hang in twos when they grow. Figs increase the motility of **male sperm** and increase the numbers of sperm cells to overcome male sterility.

Grapefruits, Oranges, and other **Citrus** fruits look just like the **mammary glands.**

Onions look like **body cells**.

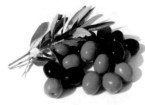

Olives assist the health and function of the **ovaries**.

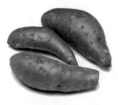

Sweet Potatoes look like the **pancreas**

"Take these steps to cut diabetes risk"

By Barbara Quinn
MCT News Service/*San Diego Union-Tribune*
July 8, 2008

Every 21 seconds someone is diagnosed with diabetes ...

... we learned from the American Diabetes Association last month at its 68th Scientific Sessions in San Francisco.

This meeting of researchers, clinicians and educators had two things in mind – how to prevent and treat the worldwide epidemic of diabetes.

Besides a huge pile of papers and products to review when I get home, here are some numbers I remember:

Eat between 25 and 38 grams of dietary fiber a day. Various natural fibers in legumes, lentils, whole grains, vegetables and fruits have been found to reduce the risk for developing type 2 diabetes by as much as 24 percent to 45 percent, we were told by Janet King, Ph.D. And we "are doing pathetically at getting fiber into the U.S. population," Julie Miller, Ph.D. added.

If you are overweight, do what you can to lose at least 10 percent of your weight. Even a modest amount of weight loss, said many experts at this conference, can help lower blood glucose, blood pressure and blood cholesterol levels – major risk factors for diabetes.

Get a pedometer and walk 10,000 steps a day. (That's about five miles.) More than one top diabetes researcher told us that increased physical activity is an important key to preventing and treating type 2 diabetes – the form most related to excess weight. Tricia (my roommate at the conference) and I had an "unofficial" competition as we counted our steps to and from the conference each day. Hint: Fidgeting in meetings and taking the stairs instead of the escalator go a long way to logging extra steps.

Limit television/computer game time to less than 10 hours a week. That's how we'll find the time to get our 10,000 steps a day. And it's one of the strategies proved to help prevent weight gain, according to researcher Rena Wing, Ph.D.

Cut the sugar. The average American consumes 30 teaspoons of sugar a day, said registered dietitian Hope Warshaw. And much of that comes from sodas and other sweetened beverages. The jury is still out on how sweetened beverages affect our risk for diabetes. But it doesn't take a diabetes scientist to realize that those liquid calories we routinely slug down only add to our national waistline.

Find ways to manage stress in your life. Rats that are stressed seek out high fat and high sugar "comfort foods" that ultimately cause weight gain, according to researcher Mary Dallman, Ph.D.

Calculate your bone health. (Diabetes increases your risk for osteoporosis and bone fractures.) One of the speakers told us about this cool online fracture risk assessment tool developed by the World Health Organization; Visit shef.ac.uk/FRAX.

Log on to sites that help you prevent and manage diabetes. Here are two: diabetes.org (American Diabetes Association) and diabetescontrolforlife.com, a free Web site that helps you plan menus, find recipes, take a portion control quiz and find other helpful tools to manage diabetes.

Stay tuned. We have more knowledge and tools than ever before to prevent and control diabetes.

* * * * * * * * * * * * * * * * *

Diabetes increases your risk for osteoporosis and bone fractures.

"Watermelon: A treat any way you slice it"

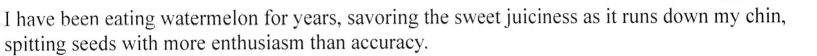

By Jeff Mullin, Senior Writer
The Enid News & Eagle (Okla.)
July 5, 2008

Wow. Watermelon. Who knew?

I have been eating watermelon for years, savoring the sweet juiciness as it runs down my chin, spitting seeds with more enthusiasm than accuracy.

I never knew I was actually ingesting a form of veggie Viagra.

That's the word, at least, from a group of scientists in Texas. They have found watermelons contain an ingredient called citrulline, which can spark production of a compound that helps relax the body's blood vessels.

That is similar to the effect Viagra has on the male, er, anatomy.

The compound, arginine, has other beneficial effects, as well. It can help heart patients with angina, can lower high blood pressure and can assist with other cardiovascular problems.

Watermelon. Wow. Who knew?

Of course to boost the body's level of arginine, you would have to eat about six cups of watermelon to get the proper amount of citrulline. Anyone eating watermelon to improve his love life should take into consideration the side effects of ingesting that much watermelon.

First, you will have to spend a great deal of time in the bathroom, given that a watermelon is mostly water. Also, watermelon contain a great deal of sugar. Putting that much sugar into your bloodstream all at once could cause cramping, which could certainly put a crimp in a guy's, er, amour.

Actually, you can get much more citrulline from watermelon rind than you can from the flesh, but who wants to eat that stuff? It also is present in cucumbers and cantaloupe, but at lower levels.

So watermelon is your best bet to obtain citrulline, a fact that should not be overlooked by those who grow and market melons.

The National Watermelon Promotion Board bills watermelon as "healthy and delicious, every day." Maybe they could spice it up a bit. How about "Watermelon is for lovers," or "Watermelon, it's not just for picnics anymore." OK, maybe not.

Watermelon isn't the only food that can benefit our health, of course. The Omega-3 fatty acids in fish can help your brain, a diet containing soy can lower your risk of cancer, oranges can help support your immune system and oat bran can help lower cholesterol.

But watermelon is the only food known to man that apparently can do, you know, which puts it in a class all its own.

Marketers of drugs such as Viagra, Cialis and Levitra are likely unhappy about the discovery of watermelon's hidden power. They may be tempted to run ads pointing out the fact their products do not require slicing or the spitting of seeds.

But that is half the fun of eating watermelon. Or it was, at least, until this recent news broke. There is nothing better on a hot summer afternoon than slicing off a big hunk of a pink, juicy watermelon and sinking your teeth into it, spitting seeds and wiping juice off your chin as you go.

And despite its newfound reputation as some sort of love potion, watermelon will continue to be a staple of picnics and church socials alike, though it might be a good idea to keep your teenage daughter's boyfriend away from the stuff, just to be on the safe side.

According to the International Festival of Competitive Eating, the world record for watermelon eating is held by Jim Reeves of Buffalo, N.Y., who consumed 13.22 pounds of the stuff in 15 minutes in July 2005 at the Brookville (Ohio) Community Picnic. Whether or not Mr. Reeves experienced any, er, unusual side effects from his excessive melon consumption, is not recorded.

OK, let's try another slogan. Watermelon, don't leave home without it. OK, maybe not.
* * * * * * * * * * * * * * * * * *

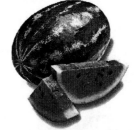
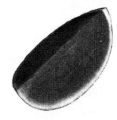

"Secret's in the Sauce"

By Caroline Dipping
San Diego Union-Tribune
July 9, 2008

Bull's-Eye Barbecue Sauce has reformulated all its sauces by removing the high fructose corn syrup, that stuff many people want to avoid because it's made from genetically modified corn and some research indicates it messes with your appetite and blood triglyceride levels.

Conducting a highly scientific test in which Bull's-Eye was squirted onto index fingers and licked clean, newsrooms tasters concluded the sauce was no worse for wear flavor-wise.

An 18-ounce bottle of the new formula retails for $2.09 in supermarkets.

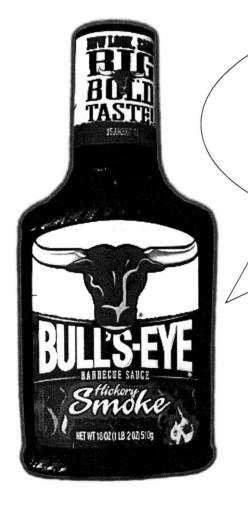

Let us hope that more food manufacturing companies reformulate their products to healthier ingredients.

* *

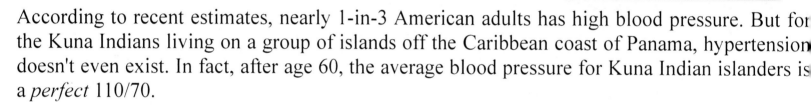

"Cholesterol drugs advised for kids with risk factors

Pediatricians group aims to forestall future heart issues"

(Author: If our children learned healthy nutrition early, these drugs may not be needed!)

By Lindsey Tanner
Associated Press/*San Diego Union-Tribune*
July 7, 2008

CHICAGO — For the first time, an influential doctors group is recommending that some children as young as 8 be given cholesterol-fighting drugs to ward off future heart problems.

It is the strongest guidance ever given on the issue by the American Academy of Pediatrics, which released its new guidelines today. The academy also recommends low-fat milk for 1-year-olds and wider cholesterol testing.

Dr. Stephen Daniels of the academy's nutrition committee said the new advice is based on mounting evidence showing that damage leading to heart disease, the nation's leading killer, begins early in life.

It also stems from recent research showing that cholesterol-fighting drugs are generally safe for children, Daniels said.

Several of these drugs are approved for use in children, and data show that increasing numbers are using them.

"If we are more aggressive about this in childhood, I think we can have an impact on what happens later in life ... and avoid some of these heart attacks and strokes in adulthood," said Daniels, a pediatrician in the Denver area. He has worked as a consultant to Abbott Laboratories and Merck & Co., but not on matters involving their cholesterol drugs.

Drug treatment would generally be targeted for kids at least 8 years old who have too much LDL, the "bad" cholesterol, along with other risky conditions, including obesity and high blood pressure.

For overweight children with too little HDL, the "good" cholesterol, the first course of action should be weight loss, more physical activity and nutritional counseling, the academy says.

Pediatricians should routinely check the cholesterol of children with a family history of inherited cholesterol disease or with parents or grandparents who developed heart disease at an early age, the recommendations say. Screening also is advised for children whose family history isn't known and for those who are overweight, obese or have other heart-disease risk factors.

Screening is recommended sometime after age 2 but no later than age 10, at routine checkups. The academy's earlier advice said cholesterol drugs should be considered only in children older than 10 after they fail to lose weight. Its previous cholesterol-screening recommendations also were less specific and did not include targeted ages for beginning testing.

Because obesity is a risk factor for heart disease and often is accompanied by cholesterol problems, the academy recommendations say low-fat milk is appropriate for 1-year-olds "for whom overweight or obesity is a concern."

The academy has long recommended against reduced-fat milk for children up to age 2 because saturated fats are needed for brain development.

"But now we have the obesity epidemic and people are thinking maybe this isn't such a good idea," said Dr. Frank Greer of the University of Wisconsin, co-author of the guidelines report, which appears in this month's edition of *Pediatrics*, the group's medical journal.

Very young children are increasingly getting fats from sources other than milk, and Greer said the updated a dvice is based on recent research showing no harm from reduced-fat milk in these youngsters.

IT'S NOT A QUESTION OF WHAT TO EAT, BUT WHAT NOT TO EAT!

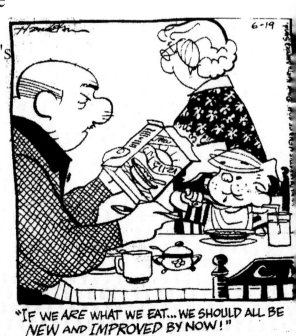

"IF WE ARE WHAT WE EAT... WE SHOULD ALL BE NEW AND IMPROVED BY NOW!"

Conclusions for a Healthy Life

We will be healthier and happier when ...

~ doctors prescribe what foods to *eliminate* from our diets, and what good foods we should eat, for our bodies' best performance and health.

~ doctors prescribe exercises appropriate for individual conditions.

~ leaders in all areas: religious, political, educators, physical trainers, all health practitioners and parents, are good examples to follow.

~ leaders learn what it takes to achieve good health and then encourage adults and children to follow these principles.

~ parents say "no" to their children's diets of sugar and flour.

~ children ask their parents for fruit rather than candy.

~ *children understand that what they learn now about nutrition, exercise, and their bodies, can give them a healthier, happier, and longer life.*

What is Happiness?
There are several definitions …

One is having enough Money, Power, Prestige, Luxury. Having a loving partner to share one's life with, and children to complete the family.

Or the love of a skill and practicing it, be it Carpentry, Music, Art, or Medicine. Of course one must begin these "Arts" by learning the theory, and then perfecting them through practice.

But even with all that, one cannot have true happiness without health. What you have learned in this book is the beginning of your path to good health.

The more you follow the eating and lifestyle plan, the more you will see less illness in your body, you will have more energy, and you will be at your best weight. Without good health, all these other material things mean nothing! In talking about something that's rarely mentioned, the "Art" of caring for the welfare of other people besides oneself.

Some say, "What's in it for me?" Well, I can tell you this, The rewards are not tangible, are not in any way Monetary gains, but can be the most exciting and Rewarding experience in your life! You will, with practice, attain this feeling, knowing that what you did helped an unfortunate person out of the dilemma he or she was in. As you learn how to eat right and get healthy, you can help others by sharing this knowledge. Just think how you could help many people by being an example. You will show them how they too can lose weight, heal certain diseases, and be healthier than they ever were. When you help others, and think of their needs as being more important than your own, you will be rewarded in more ways than you ever imagined.

You will then know true happiness.